The Blue Line

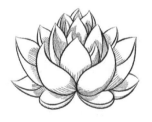

EMMA WEAVER

DEDICATION

To those who find themselves faced with fertility challenges, you are not alone

ACKNOWLEDGEMENTS

To my three children you are my world.

I am so proud to be you mum. You are my inspiration.

Chloe, I am in awe of the beautiful strong woman that you are.

Rhys, you are a beautiful soul with an amazing future.

Amelia, you have completed our family and are

such a joy in all of our lives. Just be you.

Mum and Dad thank you for giving me wings

while always holding a safety net.

To all my brothers and sisters, thank you.

Karen my forever supporter,

with a bond thousands of miles couldn't break, thank you.

Niall, thank you for the journey and the memories.

Rock chicks, for your encouragement and support.

Contents

Chapter 1

My Secret

I'm lying on the yoga mat wondering how I got to this point. Where is the feisty, powerful young woman who used to be there? I hardly recognise myself in the mirror. Yoga is my favourite place to be. Lying on the mat at the end of a session meditating my life into order. Breathe in for seven and out for eleven. In for seven and out for eleven. These breaths help me gain head space. Being a journalist can be so challenging, especially in a small town. Yoga gives me that clarity in my head. Right, that's enough. Back to reality. Quick shower and over to the hula hotel to meet the girls so I can be their weekly shoulder to cry on. Their lives are different to mine. They have husbands, kids, broken careers and domestic animals to care for and in their eyes, I have a dream life of no responsibilities. If only they realised. It's not that easy.

Beautiful smiles and fresh faces after yoga. We meet on a weekly basis. Cassy, a natural beauty, married with three children and living a dream life next to the sea. She has an option to stay at home but chooses not to and avails of a beautiful, toned, well-educated au pair to mind the children while she pursues her modelling career. Not bad for a mum of three.

Patrice, beautiful soul, two children, a controversial partner and a stay-at-home mum. Money is no object but a small price to pay for happiness. Never happy, always yearning and her cup is never full, but someone we all love so much.

Marie, the youngest of us all, has the world at her fingertips. Glamorous, educated, high-end job, model man and a great head on her shoulders. We love her because she reminds us of what we are missing. She cannot understand small town girls, although I imagine she loves it, really. She, the city type who always comes back. We enjoy hearing the stories of adventure and socialites in city bars.

That's the gang introduced, now for coffee and cakes. Today has been a particularly hard day. It was yet another trip to hospital to hear more bad news and those two words rocked my world to the core. 'Unexplained Fertility.' What even is that? We've spent years of trying, tests, peeing on sticks, lying upside down, legs in the air. Every book imaginable to man has been sought and read, analysed, and read again to make sure no stone is unturned on our quest for a baby. Devastation doesn't even come close. Most of all, it's our big secret.

Kiss, kiss. We are all happy to see each other and the atmosphere in the hotel is wonderful as always. Fire light, piano in the background, and the hustle and bustle of check in and late check out.

'How was yoga?'

'Fabulous as always. If I won the lotto, I would go every day.'

'How has your day been, Cassy?'

'Aw, same old same old. Photo shoot this morning and podcast this afternoon. Then home to dinners, bathing kids and homework, the joys,' Cassy says, laughing.

Life is a balancing act, and Cassy seems to balance her life very well. She knows her limits and will always delegate and employ more staff if need be or if there is a lot going on. Her children are well-educated and have impeccable manners, and the constant juggling about does not seem to faze them at all, which is great. Shelly, the au pair, does a great job keeping routine and order in the household.

Patrice is having a hard time with the school and cannot understand why no one else has picked up on the same issue in the class. The teacher is obviously not impressed with the private tuition and home schooling the children have received, and Patrice is determined the children will continue to have both. She's looking radiant in size ten jeans and top, makeup perfected, and a smile to light up a room, the woes of exercise and diet never escape her thoughts for too long. Even the latte we have just ordered has to be skinny. Hey, who are we to judge?

Marie is quiet this evening. She's driven a long way to join us for our weekly meet up and we are truly grateful, even if she is quiet. We ask if everything is all right and get a short answer so the return of the waiter with our order is greatly welcomed.

Should I tell them or not? I feel bad keeping this massive part of my life a secret, but I feel I may crumble if I tell or even be judged. It is supposed to be the most natural thing in the world to reproduce and here I am sitting after being told Keith and I can't even do that, but there are options. Yes, at least there are options.

Chapter 2

We Have Options

As I drive up the driveway, I feel a sense of dread. That lovely relaxing feeling from yoga seems a lifetime away and now I am home. The place that's supposed to be my solace is now a constant reminder the little angel I so yearn for is further away than ever. Right Sam, pull yourself together. It will work out for you. Don't let it show.

The door's open. I breathe in the lovely smell of cinnamon sticks, and dinner being cooked. Keith is such a wonderful cook. I am truly spoilt. Keith is not very good at showing his feelings. His language of love is cooking a home-cooked meal. I appreciate this so much, although going through this process can be hard and talking about it might help, especially after all these years of trying. Harry, the dog, comes racing toward me and greets me with his big puppy dog eyes and a lick that would melt your heart.

'Hello,' comes from the kitchen. 'I have cooked your favourite. Hope you're hungry.'

I am not at all hungry. My stomach is still so upset from the news, but I do not say that. Instead, I shout, 'Fantastic, I am starving. It's been a long day and I haven't had a chance to eat yet.'

We meet each other with a loving kiss and eye contact. Even after twelve years together, my heart still skips a beat. This loving man who cherishes me and would be such an amazing father has never once faltered though our trying for a baby journey. There have been many ups and downs and it has been a rollercoaster ride for sure, but we have always known we are meant to be together whatever life throws at us.

Perfect couple. So in love. When are you going to have children? Beautiful babies. This is all we hear. If only they realised. Why do people ask us all the time? They see me as a successful businesswoman depriving Keith of a child, an heir to his throne, a fulfilled life, the next generation. Little do they know. No one knows.

'Now we know what we are dealing with, we can do something about it,' are Keith's words of comfort.

We don't know what we are dealing with. They say it is unexplained. Are we genetically incompatible for having children? Should we not try? Will they be all right if we are fortunate to conceive? All these thoughts run through my head but best keep them there, in my head. I do not want to cause a fuss. Yearning for a child consumes every aspect of your life even when you don't realise it.

Breath in for seven and out for eleven. Tuesday night yoga. I am still so full of anxiety and fear that even yoga is not helping me tonight. I count the cracks in the tiles on the wall. This is bliss. My little piece of heaven, ME time. Ahh! Lying here trying to somehow meditate myself pregnant without having to choose a life without children or go through treatment.

'Sam. Sam.'

I hear a gentle whisper. My yoga teacher says the session is over. I laugh awkwardly and get up, head for a shower, put on some makeup and head to meet the girls, just what I need.

'Hey, no Marie tonight,' Cassy and Patrice say. 'She texted to say she wasn't able to make it, some prior engagement or something.'

What a beautiful evening. The hotel is situated on a lake and boasts beautiful scenic views of calm water, a jetty and islands surrounding the lake. There are boats of all shapes and sizes that glide along the water, and people taking in the last of the sunshine and a lovely autumn evening, they look so peaceful.

'So, how has your week been?' Cassy asks.

'All good,' I reply, 'well except for the normal trials and tribulations of being a journalist and having to deal with the public on a daily basis. Covering what the big news story is for that day. And ensuring everyone is happy and politically correct in their opinions. What ever happened to freedom of speech?'

There, that should be enough to deter Cassy and Patrice from asking too many questions about my week. I have become a master of diverting the conversation from me. If I were to tell them what was really happening with me, they would smother me with concern, love and kindness and that is not what I need right now. I must figure this out for myself.

'Well, enough from misery guts over there trying to change the world, wait until I tell you what has been going on in the school this week,' Patrice says. 'They have called me and Tim in to discuss the conflict of interest with the extra tutorials the children are having and recommend we stop sending them.'

'Can they do that? Cassy asks.

'No,' replies Patrice. 'But the cheek of them. The education system is so different here. They do not seem to want outside influence at all. I think they are intimidated by another qualified person shining a light on the inadequate system they have here.

The obsession on exams and academia being the only system they have to quantify a child's intelligence and skills when there are so many other ways to do this, astounds me. Anyhow, that's my rant over. No way am I giving up the children's tutor. She is a life coach also and teaches social skills, motivational thinking and mindfulness. You don't get that at school. Where is my skinny latte?'

Cassy and I laugh. 'Oh Patrice, a full latte is not going to make you fat.'

'A moment on the lips is a lifetime on the hips,' replies Patrice while she asks for some shortbread to go with her skinny latte.

Cassy is just glad to get out of the house as she hasn't been working all week and has spent it indoors with the children. Doing the school run seems to have taken its toll on her. She is rather pale looking and when we asked, she said she was suffering from exhaustion from the week of running she's had. Oh, to have money and an au pair.

'I'm home,' I shout. Closing the door behind me, I find Keith in the living room with a letter in his hand. I can tell from the brown envelope on the floor it is a hospital letter. Keith looks up.

'Well, here it is. The letter stating we are candidates for treatment, and we have an appointment for the end of the week.'

My heart stops. I am holding back tears. This is it. We can no longer fool ourselves into thinking we can achieve this on our own and now have to hand our hopes and desires to science to give us a helping hand. 'What are we going to do?' I say sitting down on the settee beside Keith, trying desperately to read his face for an emotional response of some kind. But I cannot see anything. He, too, is numb and very matter of fact.

'We go,' he says.

We listen to our options and take it from there. In the meantime, we keep doing what we are doing, and things might happen naturally. I sit, staring at the letter, punch the time and date into my google calendar and wonder how I will get the time off work.

'How was your day?' Keith asks to change the subject now we have decided to keep going.

I bring my thoughts back to the present and tell him about my woes as a local journalist. How Patrice has taken on the school and is kicking up such a fuss and how poor Cassy looked exhausted because she has been an at home mum all week. We laugh at the paradox and gently hug.

'I am starving,' says Keith. 'Fancy take out?'

'I'm always hungry.'

***

Next morning, things are the same. Alarm goes off, we get up, showered, dressed, breakfast, kiss goodbye and off to work we go. I feel so empty. The longing for a baby to complete my little family never goes away. There is not a day that goes by that I do not think about it. I really try not to let it overpower me, but I would be lying if I said it does not bother me. Most mornings, I am crying with pain in the shower. The anguish for my baby hurts my heart so much. I face each day with this secret, and no one knows, only myself and Keith. Work keeps me busy. I love my job. I am a naturally curious person and love to people watch. Journalism allows me to feed my curiosity every day and help people to tell their stories. The downside is I come from a rural area, so everyone knows me. If I get a story wrong or I am too controversial in my approach, I face a week of Chinese whispers, bad looks and angry emails. All part of the job, I suppose. Today I am travelling to a seaside town to cover a story of deception and lies. A business couple who owned a multimillion-pound export agency were found cutting corners within the factory and one apparently making more money than the other. They say money is the root to all evil and it cannot buy you happiness, yet it seems to mean so much to so many people, ruining lives, causing pain and devastation. Not just here, but all over the world. These things cross my mind and with corporate types getting richer and the poor getting poorer, you wonder where it is all going to end. As I'm a journalist, I try not to have an opinion, stick to the facts and tell the story in a factual entertaining way which can be quite hard given the task in hand. I enter the office and I'm met by some furious men and others looking on. I introduce myself and try to alleviate the tension in the room. I interview the men individually and also get some comments from staff. I put my notes in my bag and get in my car, stopping for some chips on my way home. I'm not supposed to eat chips. I am on a strict fertility diet. But hey, at this stage, after three years of trying, I don't think a bag of chips will change much.

I call into the office to write up my story and add the pictures to the piece and call in to the boss to ask for Friday morning off.

'Oh eye,' he says. 'Friday morning off can only mean one thing about here with female journalists. Is there a little one on the way? Isn't that book in at the hospital maternity clinic?' he says laughing.

Only I don't think it's funny and the expression on my face says it all. People can be so insensitive to childless couples assuming it is by choice and never thinking otherwise. I throw him off the track by saying, 'Oh great, so you're saying I look pregnant now, are you?' To which he stammers and does not know what to say. I repeat my request for Friday morning off to which he agrees. I go back to my desk feeling exhausted from all the secrets and lies. I finish my article and head out for the rest of the day, camera in hand as you never know when you could catch a story.

It is stunning where I live. I take a moment to breathe in the air and be grateful for such beauty and nature. I come from a small town that has the right balance of nature and development enough to sustain a life, work, family and connect with nature daily. I suddenly notice my surroundings and become mindful of my thoughts. It autumn and the leaves are falling from the trees. It is time to let go, to release the things that do not serve a higher purpose in our lives. Like the tree shredding its leaves to prepare for the fresh new ones that will come in spring. There may be a harsh winter in between but the new leaves in spring will be worth the struggle of winter. It is not like me to be so deep with my thoughts. I'm pretty forward thinking and process things on face value basis. I feel alive. I feel I am in the right place at the right time and that I need to shred myself of any preconceptions of fertility. I need to not concern myself of what the issue is. I need to not judge myself and Keith for not making this happen ourselves. I need to be like the autumn trees and shred what does not serve a purpose for my greater good. And I need to and brace myself for the winter struggle I am now faced with as it will all be worth it if my little bud starts to grow in spring. Suddenly, I have found the strength to cope, to understand and most of all support Keith through our journey. Right then and there I see a beautiful bird sitting looking at me with the most magnificent colours I have ever seen. I do not know what type of bird it is. All I know is that it is the sign of hope I have needed.

Chapter 3

The Journey

Friday morning, alarm goes off. It makes no difference because I did not sleep anyway. I suspect Keith did not sleep much either. Up, showered, dressed and breakfast as usual, no goodbye kiss this morning as we are both leaving together, both feeling nervous and not talking much. Ok, have we got the car keys, yep, my bag, yep, the letter for the hospital, yep. Ok then, all set, let's go. There it is, the kiss! The reassurance I have needed all morning. I can feel myself trembling inside with nerves as I do not know what to expect when we get there and how to process what is happening.

Through the doors of the state-of-the-art new hospital, busy as always, we follow the signs to our section and are greeted by a familiar face at reception. We exchange pleasantries, book in and take our seat. Excited, expectant mums and dads coming for their baby scans fill the large room. Some look pregnant and others are showing no signs at this stage. They're nervously sitting, waiting to be called so they can get the first glimpse of their little baby on the scan. Keith holds my hand as we absorb the atmosphere and wish that will be us soon.

A pleasant nurse calls us in. We meet with the consultant doctor. He sits me down beside him and Keith on a different seat away from us. I can see the discomfort in Keith's face. The consultant asks the same questions they have asked us several times by now. How long have we been trying for a baby? When was my last menstrual cycle? How long are they? Family history. All the test results are in that Keith and I have done. Given our age and healthy lifestyle, it was hard to pinpoint exactly what the cause of our infertility is, and we now need to discuss options.

A referral is being made to attend the fertility clinic in the main hospital in our nearest city. This is the only place that provided treatment, and the waiting list starts at two years. It is advisable to consent to being added to the list now as the wait is so long. Oh, my word! Two years! I can feel the tears coming to my eyes. Why is it so long? So not only do you have to wait to be unsuccessful in conceiving for two years, we now have to continue trying and wait another two years.

'Yes,' the consultant explained. 'There is a long waiting time due to the enormity of the problem here.'

He tries to reassure me that things will be happening within those two years. We will attend appointments, screening and monitoring of our health, which is of no comfort to me. I look at Keith and he appears as equally upset about the news as I am, so I pull myself together and decide to do this logically. Ok right, what do we do now? I again have to go for another intrusive test, then blood tests and urine samples. Keith then has to give blood also which is funny as he does not like this at all. He had better get used to it because we are in for a long ride. We sign consent papers and leave sticky-plastered and feeling a bit deflated. What a rollercoaster. We get in the car.

'Let's go for coffee,' Keith said.

I love going for coffee with Keith. We both have such busy lives separate to each other through work and other commitments. Coffee is a bit of our time together publicly to remind ourselves and others that yes, we do have a partner. I am so proud to have Keith on my arm and it just feels right. We chat about silly things, the smell of the coffee, people we meet, what to do at the weekend and gossip a little about work. It is just so nice to get out, breath and be Sam and Keith, not the journalist or the lecturer and certainly the couple desperately trying to have a child. I can see how people get lost in the process as it is all-consuming even when you don't want it to be. As we part ways for the afternoon, I ponder what to do for the weekend. I am not pondering too long when my phone beeps to remind me it is Cassy's birthday on Sunday, and this can only mean one thing. GIRLS NIGHT! This couldn't have come at a better time and I group chat with Cassy, Patrice and Marie to see what the plans are. Actually, that's strange, we haven't made any already as it is tomorrow night. Perhaps I have been too occupied in my own stuff, I have forgotten.

After many texts and debate what to do, we settle for a very sensible meal and few drinks. Gone are the days of nightclubs and all-nighters. Birthdays used to be messy, but with poetry class and choir on a Sunday morning, the girls want to be on top form. In fact, Cassy will drive, and it's her birthday. Now what to wear? I need a distraction after my long week, months, years even, so a night out is just what I need.

Saturday night came and went, and a lovely Sunday morning lie in with my hubby. I am feeling a little fragile after the night before and being spoilt by Keith is just heaven. It was great to catch up with the girls and feel young again. The food was awesome, and a few glasses of wine did me the world of good. I have been so careful over the years about what I eat and drink to increase my fertility; I have decided not to be so hard on myself. Keith is the same. He has been on a strict fertility diet, no tight underwear. He has even tried acupuncture and Chinese medicine that looked like muck from the garden. Oh, when I think about what we have tried, what we have eaten and how hard we have prayed to conceive, and it appears it is not to be. Still, I keep the secret. I will not let anyone in. It is too hard. We don't want sympathy. And we don't want questions or even help. We just want a baby, our baby.

***

Tuesday night yoga. Ahh bliss, lovely tranquillity, some time to relax, revive and meditate. The instructor is amazing, and it is an all-female class. That allows me to relax even more. I love the smell of the incense. It takes me to a different place, clears my mind and allows total calm. In for seven and out for eleven, in for seven and out for eleven. I can feel my breaths changing my thoughts and leading me into a meditative state. It is hard to relax with all the questions in my head. Why us? What can we do to increase our chances to have a baby? Maybe we are not meant to have children. My mind wanders into another head space. I need to calm down and use this time to slow down and breathe. I feel suffocated, almost with grief. In a way, I have. Every month I'd long for a positive pregnancy test, hoping not to menstruate and knowing the pain when I did. And for all those times it was late and the hope I felt only to be disappointed. Telling Keith was like ripping his heart out as he was waiting in anticipation too. It is all we talked about after deciding many years ago to start a family.

'Ok now ladies. That's it for another week.'

Up I get, shower, and off to meet the girls I go. I am not really in the mood to meet the girls this evening. I am afraid I may cry when they are chatting. I feel very raw, vulnerable and emotional. I am the last one to arrive, and the girls are there already.

'Hi, how was yoga?' They greet me before I sit down.

Ok, now I know something is up. 'All right ladies, what is it? I laugh as the waitress comes to take our order.

'Cassy has something to tell you,' Marie says.

I look at Cassy who does not seem happy at all and say, 'What is it? Is everything ok?'

'Yes,' Cassy replies, 'everything is ok. I'm just not feeling myself and now I know why. I'm pregnant, Sam,' she announces.

The girls sit in silence, looking straight at me to see what my reaction is. I jump up as quick as I can and give Cassy a massive hug and congratulate her. She appears relieved. I laugh and ask why she is so relieved.

She is embarrassed and says, 'Well, it is not planned but a welcomed surprise. We are just delighted, even though this probably means my modelling career is over and I am going to turn into a stay-at-home mom trying to fill my days,' Cassy says for dramatic effect.

We all laugh out loud because we all know that will never happen. Everyone goes silent and I am still sitting with a massive smile on my face and then Cassy breaks the silence.

'You see, Sam, we all thought that you would be next. You know, to get pregnant. Both me and Patrice have had our children or well at least we thought we had until this little surprise came along. And Marie, well Marie is too busy leading the high life to be tying herself down with children.'

Marie appears offended. 'I would love to have kids. I would be a great mum.'

I look at the girls and their faces edged with sympathy and I declare, 'Ladies, motherhood is just not for me, not yet at least. I have a career to consider and opportunities to pursue it is just not on the cards for me yet.'

At least it wasn't all lies.

'Well, that's ok then,' states Patrice and everyone relaxes.

I laugh, and the intensity subsides. Everyone assumes you want children. Childbearing age is a strange time for women. What if I didn't want children? I know I do, and I am trying, but they don't know that. The looks of sympathy on their faces even without knowing our struggle is the exact reason I have not told them. I have not told anyone.

'I'm home,' I shout as I close the door behind me. Keith greets me in the hall.

'Hi, how was your day?'

'Grand,' I reply. 'Is that lasagne I smell? Mmm.'

Keith laughs. 'It sure is.'

As I walk to the kitchen, I decide just to tell Keith Cassy's news instead of sitting in silence. 'Cassy's pregnant,' I say in a high pitch tone trying to sound ok about it and without my voice cracking.

'Oh,' Keith replies, 'that's nice.'

'Mmm, you knew,' I say. 'I can tell by your relaxed tone.'

I should have guessed something was amiss. As always, Keith's language of love is food. When he is not dealing with an emotion or he knows I am finding things difficult, he cooks.

'Yes, I did. Cassy wanted to tell you herself. I was chatting to James outside work. He is a bit stunned but happy. He had not expected to be a dad to four kids. Three was his limit.'

'Poor James,' I said laughing, trying to joke about it. 'How do you feel Keith?'

He shrugs his shoulders, and says, 'It is what it is. How are you?'

I shrug mine and say, 'Another birth won't make a difference. Since we started trying to conceive, five babies have been born between both our families and another one will not make any difference. I don't care about anyone having a baby and I genuinely mean that. I don't want their baby. I want our baby. There is a massive difference. I don't feel jealous or envious. It is not my baby. I just want our baby.'

Keith gives me a big hug, making me feel he doesn't believe me.

'Oh, now I get it. That's why you made lasagne,' I announce. Keith laughs, and we sit down to eat, still with love in our eyes and a glimmer of hope. A cosy evening at home with a fire blazing, our dog on the mat and a documentary on the television.

***

Beep, beep, beep! Alarm goes off. Up I rise, shower, breakfast, kiss goodbye and out the door. I enjoy routine. It helps me to stay focussed and feel ready for anything. Today's story is one of tragedy—a local lad killed on a bad stretch of road. Local residents are calling the council to resurface the road. It is a public consultation meeting and they always tend to be heated. At least I am not on camera duty today. The paper has allocated a photographer. That always makes life easier. I am not good at taking photographs, it's not my forte.

People take tragedy so differently. Some people feel sad, grieve quietly and revert into themselves. Others still get out and about and appear sad. Then there are others who are proactive and seek to actively change things or divert the grieving process by becoming an activist. I love people watching. People and their behaviours fascinate me. Everyone deals with things in their own way, and that's ok. There is no right or wrong way so long as no one gets hurt.

Home is a little strange at the moment. We are talking and communicating but holding back a little, trying to see how the other is feeling. We are waiting with anticipation for our next appointment though it could be awhile, especially as there is a two-year waiting list. Who knew things were that bad? Why is there such an issue with fertility? Especially in young couples. Is it the water? Is it the food we are eating? Colouring our hair? What is it? I have researched this for years and tailored both my lifestyle and Keith's lifestyle habits. No alcohol, proper food, long walks, exercise, loose clothes, vitamins, zinc, hopi candles, acupuncture. You name it; we have tried it. It is soul destroying trying to conceive. Month in and month out hoping and praying for the first signs of early pregnancy, recording body temperature, urinating on ovulation sticks. Only making love on favourable days, which takes the whole romance from your relationship and it becomes so medicalised and controlled. We always enjoyed a healthy sex life and are very attracted to each other, so to control things and not be as free with each other definitely brought a different light to our relationship. The intrusive assessments and questions the doctors and consultants ask are out of this world embarrassing but shows the strength of our relationship. There have definitely been some embarrassing moments and some really funny ones. You just have to remember what you are doing this for and forget everything else. After all, we still have to look at each other and fancy each other and respect our relationship.

After work, I head home, still taking in the day's events and the outrage at the public meeting. It makes a good story, but it is awful how tragedy affects people's lives, whole generations affected by events. I stop by the shop and pick up something nice for dinner. I thought I better show a bit of an effort as Keith works hard too.

When I get home, the house is quiet. I shout hello, but there's no answer. I throw my keys on the hall table, put my coat and bag on the hanger and look around for Keith. I eventually find him sitting outside in the backyard, on the bench, freezing, smoking a cigarette.

'Keith,' I yell. 'What are you doing? You don't smoke, not anymore anyway.'

Keith looks at me and I know not to say anything more, the stress is all over his face. This is it. I think he has had enough. He has been so strong for so long. He has had enough, and he's throwing in the towel. I sit down beside him. He politely puts the cigarette out, looks at me and speaks.

'I can't do it.'

My heart sinks right to my toes and on to the ground. I feel the tears coming to my eyes. *Do I speak or not?* I need to plead, *please, don't give up, please.* My head is spinning. I don't know where to start.

When Keith speaks again, he says, 'I can't do it. I can't wait two years.

Then, just like that, we talk about going private, finding the money and we dare to dream that this all might happen for us sooner than we realise. I feel empowered and back in control of my life, my future, and there is hope again. That evening we didn't cook. The fire was lit, a takeaway was ordered, and we shared some wine. We spent the evening giddy and laughing at the possibilities of having a baby, how our lives would change and how much we would love to become parents. Keith spoke of the shame and guilt he felt as a man not being able to reproduce, the most natural thing in the world and he could not do it. He explained it made him feel less of a man and he feared I would leave. I'd been so busy processing my own feelings and sense of being a failure as a woman, I did not realise Keith was having similar thoughts. The feeling of shame I did not relate to, and Keith explained he felt his peers and others would judge him if he were to confide in anyone about our fertility issue. There is a stigma attached to infertility, and it remains very taboo, and for that reason, we decided not to tell anyone. So still I hide the secret, only now there is more to it.

Where do we start? The internet is our only means of information at this stage to find out where is available for us to have a consultation, to see how we can go forward and what our options are. My head is spinning, but in a good way. There is a lot of information to go through. As a journalist it should be no bother to me, though it seems harder when it is personal.

The day starts as normal alarm goes off, up washed, dressed and breakfast only there is a different atmosphere in the house. Keith doesn't feel so helpless now that we have decided to go private.

Chapter 4

Private

Appointment day. It's a long drive in the car, we are both nervous. We chat the way down the road about what the appointment might entail, the tests, different outcomes, money and time off work. Mostly it was speculation and guessing.

When we arrive, we are forty minutes early. Keith takes a phone call. I feel more nervous. I don't understand why as it is only a consultation we do not even know if there are options for us. The room is clinical. There are lots of leaflets, books. A coffee machine in the corner that you would need a degree to work it. Keith cannot help himself and decides he needs a coffee. It's a distraction, I suppose. I read the literature on the table. The receptionist comes in and asks us to fill out our details. She explains the consultant will be available soon. Another couple enter and sit in the waiting area. They call us in to see the consultant. The nurse introduces herself and guides us down a long corridor with several doors to walk through. We shake hands and take a seat. We explain our situation and the findings of investigations so far and give the documents to the consultant. Unexplained fertility, where do you even start? We are back at the beginning. The consultant wants us to go through all the tests again for their team to assess. I can't believe it as we have done them before, and they are very intrusive. It is a strange feeling. You do not want the tests to find anything and yet if they did, you would know what you are dealing with.

'Up on the bed, please.'

The nurse comes in to ensure I am comfortable, and for legal reasons I assume it is statutory to have a nurse. Curtains drawn; it is strange knowing Keith is the other side of the curtain. Beforehand, he was always out of the room.

They bring Keith down the corridor to dispense for his investigations and we go back to the consultant. He is a nice man and spends a lot of time with us and explains all the different scenarios and outcomes. He gives us plenty of literature and information and prices of treatments. There are so many types, though we cannot decide until we know our options. But for now, we know we have to pay for consultation and admin fees and the process has begun.

On the way home, we discuss the information they gave us. We stop at a retail park and find a restaurant to get something to eat before the long journey home. There is so much to consider, so many outcomes and a lot of appointments to see us through this. Financially, we will need a loan as it is expensive though this is only a minor detail at this stage as having a baby is all we can focus on. We look at each other in the restaurant knowing that this is it. This is the beginning of our treatment journey. We are confident a treatment option will be available to us based on the results of our initial consultation in our local hospital. And we've already dealt with the pain and upset of knowing that something is not right. We have been screened and tested and prodded at before and the results were not good. So as far as we're concerned, these results will be the same. Call it naivety or just knowing, we felt like we know whatever the results will be so that is not our concern. Our thoughts are on the practicality of the treatment, and which treatment option is for us. We have an appointment for next week to find out results and discuss treatment. We dare to dream that all it takes is four to five months from start to finish and we could be pregnant by spring. This thought fills us with happiness and hope. I am so glad we went private. I feel time is ticking for us, well, me really.

***

The next day we get up as always. I'm feeling a little more tired than usual. The journey up and down to the private clinic is very draining, especially in autumn when the weather is dark. Its Tuesday and the day the print run is done for the paper. With me being off yesterday, I have so much to do and start to feel the pressure of trying to juggle everything. I will take it in my stride. As long as no one knows, it will be ok. I can hold my head. I am pleased with my articles this week. They were particularly interesting, and we got some great photographs. I feel proud as I really enjoy my work.

Yoga this evening is just what I need and a catch up with the girls afterwards is overdue too. It is not that I don't want to tell the girls about what is going on. It is just Keith and I agreed not to as it then becomes all-consuming. There would be too many questions and we don't know all the answers, so it is just less complicated no one knows, even our family.

Yoga was bliss as always and I am now sitting with the girls. We are all here tonight. That has not happened in a while. Skinny lattes, cappuccinos and an herbal tea for me. Back to all this. Apparently too much caffeine is bad and if we're doing this, Keith and I doing it right. The girls do not pass remarks as they are used to me and my fad diets. At least, that's what I tell them. The chat is good. Cassy looks fabulous. She is truly blooming. Although she complains a lot about being pregnant, she has a sparkle in her eye that tells me she is so excited. I am sure it is tough if you have morning sickness and the school run to do. Patrice is busy telling her about remedies that will help with morning sickness, and tales of pregnancies that have come before, erupt.

And at that, Marie blurts out, 'I'm pregnant too.'

There is complete silence and we all sit waiting to hear more but nothing more comes from Marie's mouth. Cassy jumps up to congratulate Marie, but Marie refuses the gesture.

'Don't bother,' she says, 'I will not be keeping it. I cannot have a baby. I would not cope, and neither would Will. We have decided it is not happening. We are too young and focussed. Besides, we would have nothing to offer a baby. I'm just telling you all because you are my dear friends, but I do not want or need your advice.'

It breaks my heart. Marie looks so vulnerable and scared. This explains why she has been so quiet lately. I get up out of my seat, give Marie a huge hug and say, 'Thank you for sharing this and we will support you whatever you decide. Life has a strange way of throwing twists and turns and if nothing else, if we can't be here for each other, then what's the point?'

Patrice and Cassy just sit looking at Marie and don't say much. I think they are more in shock. I'm sure they are not judging Marie. At least, I hope not. I give them both a look as if to say come over here and show support to which Patrice does and Cassy doesn't. Cassy then pleads with Marie.

'Marie, are you sure? I think you would make a great mum. Imagine our little ones growing up together. I didn't expect to get pregnant. I didn't want any more but look how it has turned out. I'm fine and we are all happy for the new addition.'

'It is ok for you, Marie replied. 'You are married, you have money and sure you even have help. I do not have any of that. No, it's not happening. We have decided it is not the right time for us. Perhaps in a few years, but not now. I don't even know how this happened. We are so careful, but it has, and we will deal with it. I hope you understand and please do not make me regret telling you all. I just couldn't keep it a secret.'

We continue to talk. We stay longer than usual, trying to offer more support to Marie. Cassy stays quiet at the end of our meet up. I agree to meet Marie the following day for coffee.

'I'm home,' I shout.

'Hi,' Keith replies. 'We are in here.'

'We?' I reply as I enter the kitchen. There I find Keith with Adam, his high school friend.

'Look who has called round.'

'Aw hi, Adam.' We exchange hugs and smiles. 'What brings you here?' I say and they both look at me laughing to say can he not call round? We all laugh, and I ask, 'What's for tea? I'm starving.'

Adam says, 'Oh eye, eating for two, are you? It's about time you two got your act together.'

Keith and I glance at each other. Such an awkward moment. Keith quickly changes the subject. You can feel the tension in the air.

'Chicken curry,' Keith says. 'That's what's for dinner.'

Mmm. I excuse myself to go to the bathroom to freshen up before dinner. My heart is racing. I feel sick. I don't know why because it's not the first time we have been asked when we will start a family. Perhaps it is the events of the whole day and with yesterday it is all getting a bit much. I need to stay calm and focussed and not get upset or annoyed. Adam didn't mean any harm. He doesn't even know we have been trying. I go back down the stairs and join the guys. All is forgotten, and they are too busy playing the Xbox to even notice I am there. Dinner was delicious as always, and the mood much lighter. I am sure people wonder if we will ever have children. My word, we wonder that ourselves, but they are insensitive and why people think they should even comment on it baffles me. Do they even stop to think perhaps it's not that easy?

Emma Weaver

Chapter 5

Appointment time

Back down the road again, I have a feeling by the end of this we will know these roads backwards. Sitting in the waiting room again, more coffee for Keith. I think it is a nervous thing. I have a feeling we will see a lot of this place over the next while. The nurse calls us, and we walk back down the long corridor through all the doors to the consultant's room. He is not there yet and we go in and wait. I breathe in a nervous sigh, and Keith touches my hand for reassurance.

'Hello Sam, hello Keith. How are you?' the consultant asks.

We both reply, 'We are good, thanks.'

'Ok, I have your test results back and they are pretty much as predicted. There are a few minor issues but nothing that cannot be helped along. We now need to discuss your options. Fortunately, at this stage I do not think a donor is necessary. I feel we can successfully obtain pregnancy ourselves using artificial insemination or IVF as you may be more familiar with. It is a procedure called ICSI to be more precise where we take the sperm and inject it directly into the egg. We will take no chances and place it there ourselves. I feel as your consultant that this is the best treatment plan for you both and will have a higher chance of success.'

'Ok, so we are going for a procedure called ISCI?'

'Yes.'

'Is this IVF?'

'Yes, it is similar in the way we collect eggs and sperm from each partner. In conventional IVF, the sperm and eggs are mixed together in a dish and the sperm fertilises the egg naturally. In ICSI, we bypass that, and we inject the sperm directly into the egg, ensuring this takes place. It is our preferred method for your treatment, ok? All these technical terms are hard to understand, and I would rather you asked me questions than use a search engine and come up with several meanings.'

'Ok, so what will happen today? I ask.

'The nurse will take you into the treatment room and take some details and do some tests, blood samples and BMI to ensure that you are suitable candidates for treatment. We will start the planning process from there.'

We leave the room and go to the nurse's room where we both have our bloods checked, which is funny. Keith does not like needles and hates even sitting watching me get my blood taken, which is becoming a frequent observation of his. Our BMI is then checked, and they ask us many questions. Have we had treatment before? Have we had any operations? When was my last period? How frequent are they? Do I bleed after sex? All inhibitions are left at the door during this journey. We had to sign about twenty pages of consent for everything, even to allow for treatment or storage of any embryos we achieve to be used if one of us dies. Oh, my goodness, what an awful thought. We are asked if we will donate any surplus embryos to science so they can use them for studies.

Back down the road we stop at the same restaurant, lots to talk about and discuss. After leaving the nurse, the next course of action is to wait for my period, to which I then phone the clinic to tell them it has started. Then we book appointment from there. As I have just completed menstruating, it will be a whole month to wait and then go back for our treatment plan. We are having medicalised treatment, which means the treatment will control when I ovulate. This will allow for accurate embryo transfer during the peak time for successful implantation. There is so much to take in and the treatment plan looks so complicated. What if I mess up or forget? Injections! There are so many injections! I am not even sure I can do this.

Don't panic, Sam, and breathe.

Keith can see the fear in my eyes, but I don't want to talk about it as it makes me worse. So, after years of hoping my period does not come, I am now watching and waiting for it to come so we can start the treatment plan What a rollercoaster!

***

I have met with Marie a few times now as I feel so bad for her. She is so adamant she is not keeping the baby and has contacted agencies that can fulfil her wishes. It is Will who is now undecided. Marie now feels cheated as they'd agreed the best decision was not to keep it. Cassy is now not talking to Marie or at least avoiding her, which I can understand too as she is pregnant and hormonal. Not that I would know about that, but I am only assuming. Life is not so black and white, and every person has a different set of circumstances. We cannot judge people. Everyone has the right to live the life they choose that is best for them. Though to be honest, things are so up in the air for me at the moment I could do with some calm within the group. Everyone has their stuff going on. Even Patrice is having a hard time at the school with the teachers and she is thinking of taking the children out of school that would be hard. I need calm and no stress, so I feel a walk is needed. Perhaps Keith will come to. Keith is not particularly fond of walks, but he indulges me, recognising I am a little stressed.

'I must call to see Mum,' I tell him. I am avoiding Mum at the moment because she might pick up on something and then I will have to lie to her too. It's hard enough keeping secrets from the girls. We walk for a mile, breathing in the fresh air and taking in our surroundings. We both agree that when we are going through our treatment process, we need to stay away from negativity and stress. There is no point going through all the treatment to let outside influences affect the outcome. Women are very hormonal creatures and stress and upset may affect my body so I promise Keith I will consciously stay away from stress. I haven't even told Keith about Marie. Perhaps now is not the time. I need my friends around me for support even though they do not realise I still need the normality of our Tuesday night chats.

***

The day has arrived. I have started to menstruate, and I phone the clinic to confirm. The lady was pleasant and made an appointment for Keith and I to attend our treatment plan meeting. She informs me this will take about two hours, so I know this means a full day off work. They won't like this one bit and it's a Monday, the worst day to take off. Keith is glad to hear there is movement. He is a practical kind of guy and likes to feel he is sorting out our issue.

At the appointment we receive boxes of injections, Menopur, Cetrotide and Ovitrelle. My goodness, the needles look big and we have to mix them up ourselves. I have no idea. The nurse goes through the whole procedure and takes out a piece of apparatus for me to practice injecting. She tells me two fingers from my belly button is the best place to inject. I practice a few times on the object and stop because no matter how often I practice, it will not help me do it. We sit down and go through the treatment plan. It is set out nicely in a chart printed from the computer, from day one to seventeen, so I focus. Ok, seventeen days at the most and this will be all over. *You can do this, Sam.*

Keith is looking at me as though he's thinking, 'I hope you are taking all of this in because I am lost.'

The nurse tries to include us both though doesn't do a great job, and ultimately, it is my responsibility to do it right and not mess up. I feel a huge pressure to get this right as it's so important to achieve a positive outcome. At the same time, I am excited to get started, full of hope and expectation that if all goes well, we will achieve a pregnancy. That would be a dream come true.

We don't stop at the restaurant on the way home as the meds have to be refrigerated. We hadn't anticipated this, and we are starving the whole way home. That, on top of feeling tired and a little anxious, does not make a good car journey home. We both laugh at each other, acknowledging our moods, and just get on with the journey. We order a takeaway as it will be the last for a while, head straight home and put all the meds in the fridge except the ones to be kept at room temperature. If anyone comes to visit, they will see the contents of the fridge and be wondering what is going on. We are so tired by the time we get home and have a bite to eat. We discuss work and the days we'll need off and some of them we will not know about until the day before. Depending on how well my body reacts to the injections and stimulates my ovaries, we have an appointment on the fifth day of injections for a scan. We will know then when we have to go back. Keith suggests I take the week off as it will be too much hassle and stressful to keep asking for random days. I think about his suggestion and agree I will request a week off in the morning. An early night, I think. It has been a long day with much to think about. My head is spinning. I have researched the internet, joined forums, asked questions and read a lot. I am not sure how helpful this has been but if anything, it has prepared me for the worst. And all suggestions are welcome when it comes to injecting my tummy. The injection is very stingy apparently and some people suggest putting ice on the site before injecting. Some people get their partners to do it and others suggest lying flat. I suppose I should just see how I go.

***

Tuesdays are busy with work as it is the paper run day, but also the most relaxing in the afternoon. Once everything is done, we have a team meeting to regroup and decide the direction of the following week's print. After the meeting, I call into the boss's office and ask for Friday off and the following week. I know it is short notice, I explain, but I need it. Something important has come up I can't explain now. After sitting through the talk on policy and procedure, I am granted the time off. I am glad to get it as it will allow me to travel up and down to the clinic hassle free from work. My fear is it will bore me, and I'll have too much time to think about what is happening. I need a distraction. I will plan my week and keep myself busy. Cassy is off work at the moment because of her pregnancy and I can call to visit Mum like I said I would. Yes, that's it. I will plan ahead.

'You appear distracted,' the yoga teacher suggests.

I smile and say, 'Long day at work,' to pass her off. If I can't hide it from the yoga teacher, I will be useless with the girls. Over at the hotel I am the first to arrive. I grab us a seat and before I have a chance to take off my coat, Marie arrives.

'Hi.'

We hug and sit back down. 'How have you been Marie? Sorry I haven't been in touch the past few days. I've had something on.'

'I'm ok,' she replies. 'Please don't apologise. You have been a great support to me through all of this. Ah, here come the girls as I see Patrice and Cassy coming through the door.'

They come over straight away. Cassy is blooming, and I tell her this. She smiles and is thankful for my comment. As we all sit,

Marie announces she has something to tell us. We're expecting Marie to explain she is no longer pregnant, and we are all shocked to hear she is. Will has reassured her they can do this and that it is the right time for them. He always wanted to be a young dad as his parents waited until they were older to have children and he always felt the age. We are all delighted and jump up and cause a scene congratulating her. Cassy is especially delighted. Marie explains she couldn't have gone through life looking at Cassy's baby knowing her baby would have been the same age and due to hit all the same milestones.

'You will not be on your own,' we assure Marie, and we all offer to baby-sit to allow her to remain in the lifestyle to which she is accustomed. We laugh and giggle the rest of the evening. I phone Keith to say I am eating out and will be home a little later, that we are celebrating. With all the excitement in the background, I tell him Marie is expecting. Keith is a little confused why I am so happy as he thought I may feel sad because of our circumstances, but he does not realise the whole story. I decide not to go into it. It is wonderful to celebrate new life. It never makes me feel bad when others have babies. That's their baby. I want my own, not theirs. It just does not affect me that way.

Chapter 6

Being Brave

Ok, so here it goes. As instructed on my treatment plan schedule, I start the injections. I feel very nervous, Keith even more so. I read the instructions time and time again and decide to just go for it. We have a deal. Keith will draw up the injection, and I will administer it. This bit I am finding really hard, inflicting myself with pain. It really is mind over matter. I have tried so many techniques to mindfully breathe through the process. I have the ice at hand, but I am pacing now and it's never good when I pace. I have to do this twice a day. Twice a day! Ok, here goes. I put ice on the place where I will inject. I pinch the skin. Keith hands me the injection and looks on anxiously while I push the injection through. I think I was a bit forceful as it really hurt and now it stings. Eek! Keith rubs my back, gives me a kiss and heads off to work. I boil the kettle, make some tea, and turn the television on. I never watch daytime television. In fact, the television is never on much as we are both at work all week and we sit in the kitchen in the evening.

I busy myself all day catching up and tidying the house. I google more IVF and ICSI information and overload myself with too much. I receive a phone call from the clinic to confirm my appointment in two days to scan me to see if I am ovulating and how the follicles are growing. They count and measure them. This helps to know when they are ok for the egg transfer. There is so much more to all of this than we had anticipated, but I will not stress, and I will take each day as it comes and each injection at a time. I cannot let overwhelm me or take over my thinking. I have arranged to visit Mum tomorrow. Perhaps I will bring her shopping. I will see how I feel. It was a long day about the house even though it is sparkly clean. Even Keith mentions it which is a bad sign of how unkempt it was. We eat before the injection and talk about doing it at the same time every day. This is for two reasons. One, so we are clear when it is and know to be together and two, we feel it would be more effective to have them at the same time. After dinner, Keith draws up the injection. My tummy is still red from this morning. As suggested by the nurse, I will alternate right and left for the injections. You can inject into your thigh, but I have decided to do it into my tummy. In my head this makes sense, mind you, it probably makes no difference. Ice out, I give it a rub, pinch, and this time go slowly to which the injection is much harder to get through and stings me a little more than this morning.

'I can't do this,' I sob. Keith just looks at me. He runs me a bath. There is nothing he can do. I'm sure he feels a bit helpless. I can't help how I feel. It's so hard injecting myself. I lie down after, feeling very sorry for myself. Why does it have to be so hard? Why could things not just go our way? All I can think about is injecting myself in the morning. I cannot let this consume my every thought. It will drive me insane. The next morning, I wake with a whole new attitude. It's only an injection. Two seconds does it. I've been through worse, and without doing this, there will be no baby. I need to get on with it.

***

Alarm goes off, up, showered, dressed, breakfast and now injection. Keith draws it up. I don't bother with the ice. I close my eyes and just firmly stick it in. Yes, it is sore and yes, it stings but that's it, over. My poor wee tummy looks so raw. I look up at Keith, smile and say, 'There, that's that done.' He smiles and gives me a 'well done' kiss and heads to work. I wait a while before I phone Mum to head out for the day.

I drive to Mum's feeling optimistic and proud of myself and my new kick IVF butt attitude. It is a cold day so Mum may not go out, so I will stay for tea instead. Mum lives in a modest house with Dad. It's a cosy, small home, enough for the two of them to manage. Mum was an accountant and Dad a solicitor. He has not fully retired yet; he works two or three days a week keeping his hand in the business as it were. My brothers are also solicitors and they help with the family-run business. It is quite successful, and they have represented some high-profile cases. Well, local high-profile cases. As I enter the house, the usual smell of honeysuckle hits my nose. Mum loves air fresheners, and this is definitely her signature house smell.

'Hi. Kettle has just boiled,' she says. I help myself to tea and a nice wee biscuit, mmm.

'I thought we have fallen out,' Mum says.

I laugh and say, 'Oh, the busy life of a journalist. You know how it is, Mum. I am anxious. I do not feel myself. The injections are definitely affecting me. I am so bubbly and confident usually. I cannot explain the feeling. I am just all over the place, anyhow, you can always come visit me, you know. That lovely BMW sitting out the front getting rusty because you will only drive within a ten-mile perimeter.'

'The roads are not what they used to be,' Mum explains. 'There are roundabouts and traffic lights everywhere, and the amount of traffic there is on the roads, we will all die of car fumes. It's pollution that will kill us all.'

Laughing, I change the subject and ask how Dad is.

'He's fine. Why don't you stop by on your way home? He will be glad to see you. He is not that busy today.'

'Aw well see,' I say, 'depends on what we are doing. Do you fancy heading out for a while? It would be good to get out a bit of fresh air in your lungs.'

Mum is hesitant at first but eventually agrees after finishing her tea.

It is nice to have Mum out. She doesn't really go too far out of town, so I take her to the bigger town with more shops and cafes in it. We have a lovely day chatting and trying on clothes. Mum still slips me twenty pounds and tells me to get something nice. This is so unnecessary, but she insists on doing it. It's a kind of mum daughter treat thing she likes to do. After we 'shop till we drop,' we head for lunch, or afternoon tea at this time. We have had a lovely day and sit comfortably at the window of a café and order lunch. The café seems full, and more people are coming in. I feel all sweaty and uncomfortable with the crowd. I open the window for air, hoping it will reduce the feeling, but it does not. I feel shaky and uneasy. I get up. Mum looks worried and asks if I am ok. I say that I am fine. I am going to the toilet. I do not feel fine, it's a feeling I never had before, and it did not feel nice. I can only say it felt like a panic attack and it was awful. I wonder if it is a side effect of the medication. I'm not sure but make a mental note to look it up. After I compose myself, I go back out to Mum. Our lunch has arrived, so I sit down and change the subject, saying I am starving and cannot wait to eat. Mum looks at me and asks again if I am ok. I say, 'I'm grand. I forgot to eat, that's all.'

She doesn't believe me for one moment but leaves it at that. We finish lunch and have some tea and head back to the car. I am placing the bags in when I realise the time. Oh, my goodness! Look at the time! I have my injection to take, and I have to take Mum home too. Oh goodness, I will be late. What should I do? I can't take Mum back to my house because she will notice something is going on. So, I get in the car and suggest we just go straight home.

'Oh Sam,' Mum says, 'I was hoping we could call in to see your father. He would really like that.'

'Aw, another day,' I say. 'I promise.

She looks so disappointed. I hate disappointing her, but I am running late already. I cannot possibly stop. I get Mum home and rush her bags in. She offers me tea and I decline. Mum is looking at me now as if she suspects something is the matter, and something is, but I can be sure it is not what she thinks.

'I have to go now, Mum.' I give her a hug and run out the door. How did I let this happen? I have completely lost track of time. Ahh, rush hour traffic. I am really panicking now. I need to calm down. In for seven and out for eleven. In for seven and out for eleven. I feel calmer. It's ok. It will be ok. I'm not late and if the traffic continues moving, I won't be late, so keep calm. I pull up on to the drive and park behind Keith's car. I walk into the house and shout, 'Hello.' Keith is in the kitchen. He is already drawing up the injection.

'You are cutting it fine,' he says in a soft, acknowledging tone.

I agree and say, 'If only you knew, Poor Mum. Goodness only know what she thinks is going on. I just dropped her off and ran,' I laugh. Ok, pinch and jab, and there you go, another one over.

'That was not so bad,' he says. 'You're getting better at it.'

I agree and feel very proud. The injections are so hard. They sting and there are so many. I cannot see the end in sight. I have a high pain threshold but find it particularly hard to inject myself. Even though I know it's for the process and a baby is the ideal outcome, it still causes me dread. I think about it from the morning until night and even when I go to bed; I am still thinking about it. We sit down after dinner and chat about our day. I explain I had a lovely day with Mum. I mention the anxiety in the restaurant, and we try to work out if it is the injections as I have never felt that before. It didn't feel nice and I would not like to feel like that again. I run a bath and have a soak for a while. I have decided to be kind to myself for the next few weeks as I need to do this properly. It is not fair on Keith and I to go through this and not do it properly. I am trying so hard not to get stressed or upset and I will go for a walk every day to keep my circulation going. Oh, and pineapples, I must eat pineapples.

'No Mum, everything's all right. No, me and Keith didn't have a fight. I just had to do something before the shops closed,' I say, explaining why I had to rush yesterday. I hate this. Now I am actually lying to my mother to cover tracks of IVF. This does not feel good at all. Perhaps I should just hibernate.

**

Here we go again, back down the road to the clinic. Injections are going well. I am sticking to the schedule, and I discover if I chew chewing gum when injecting, it takes the edge off for me and it does not seem to sting as much. It might be in my head, but it works for me. We chat and listen to the radio, nothing too heavy, and the journey goes by quickly. We do not know what to expect at this appointment, so we are both a little apprehensive. Keith enjoys his coffee while we sit in the waiting room. A couple come in with their toddler. He is quite lively. We exchange smiles. The woman appears awkward and apologises for bringing her son to the clinic. She says it is a little insensitive. Both Keith and I assure her we do not mind in the slightest. We hadn't really thought about it. She went on then to tell us her son was an IVF baby so we should be encouraged. She said the treatment and consultants here are great with high results. This made me feel really happy and more hopeful. When you see a little boy in front of you who's been through the same process, there is something reassuring about it. I'd never thought of it like that before.

Down the long corridor and into the room. We sit waiting for the consultant. When she arrives, she explains our usual consultant is in the procedure unit today and that she will be performing the tests today. We are both happy with this. The doctor explains she will do an internal scan to see if the ovaries have been stimulated and count and measure any follicles. Oh, ok, now I understand what is happening. I go behind the curtains and have the test done and come back round to Keith.

'Everything is coming along nicely,' the doctor explains. 'Come back in three days and we will see how things are then and take it from there.'

It is such a long stretch and these injections are not the easiest thing in the world to administer. The nurse takes us into the other room to take more blood samples.

'How are things going?' she asks.

'I'm getting there. At times, I feel overwhelmed and all sweaty. I come over all strange. I do not feel like myself. I am not an anxious person, yet I feel anxious all the time. I could cry at anything and I feel slightly paranoid too. Am I going insane?' I ask the nurse.

The nurse is kind and takes the time to listen to me. I start to cry. This is the first open tear that I allow to fall down my cheek. It's so hard and the injections hurt, my heart is heavy, and my head is so full of everything. I have lost my confidence. I am so preoccupied. The nurse explains this is a process. I am full of hormones. Naturally, I will feel different and people experience things differently. She reminds me to be kind to myself, that my body is working hard, and is being controlled by a medical intervention. I agree with the nurse. I also state that being kind is definitely essential, though too much time to think takes its mental toll as my thoughts wander and do not make me feel good.

'It is all about balance,' she says. 'And oh, remember to drink plenty of water.'

I acknowledge her advice. It is one of those situations that's hard to get through, but you just have to do it. I feel strong at the moment for doing this and if it works, it will be the most amazing process. Keith and I leave and stop at the restaurant for lunch. We really are creatures of habit. We walk around the shops for a bit, messing about and trying on sunglasses and looking through fish tanks. All is well at the moment.

***

It's Marie's birthday this weekend and I can't get out of it. The only upside is that both she and Cassy are expecting so there will be no drinking for them. I might suggest an alcohol-free birthday going out in sympathy for those who cannot drink. That will get me off the hook. I could do with going nowhere as my head is spinning with these injections. I am very mindful and emotional, and my poor tummy feels awful. The next few days I keep myself to myself, communicating with others via WhatsApp or email. I am on my own little journey with this process, and I need time to myself. I go for a lovely long walk every day even though it is freezing. I head to the shops one day to buy a dress for Saturday night for Marie's birthday. A dress is my best option as it will not be sticking into my pinhole tummy. I find a lovely black dress with a flower pattern on it and treat myself to a pair of shoes too.

See Sam, it's not so bad. You have managed to get out and sort out an outfit and no anxiety or issues this time.

I head home and get ready. We are going for a meal. It was supposed to be at six, but I pushed back to accommodate taking my injection. This process takes over. Perhaps it shouldn't, but I cannot help it as it is so important. I tan myself, eyelashes on, my beautiful new dress and shoes, and I blow-dry my hair. I feel great, happy and me again.

The next day I get up, shower, dress and prepare myself for the journey to the clinic. It's another scan day today. I can definitely feel something happening in my tummy. I hope my ovaries have been stimulating and the follicles have grown. It is not so much how many we recover; it is the size of the follicles that count, I think, and poor Keith is none the wiser either. As we wait to go to the consultation room, I read up on all the literature in the waiting area. There are some interesting facts and statistics about IVF and other procedures. The statistics I don't feel are great, but I need to stay positive. The older you get, the harder it is to conceive, well for the woman anyway. We go down to the consultation room and we speak with the consultant for a few minutes, just chit chat really, and then I get up on the bed. The consultant is very pleased with my progress and counted a very high amount of follicles with several of them looking favourable. We discuss the potential of implementing the trigger injection. This is for the oocyte retrieval. It is the injection that ensures my body doesn't release the eggs that have built up in my ovaries before the egg collection. It is all so clinical and I feel like my body is just a piece of meat or an object where its main use is to grow and incubate a baby. Clinical is the right word, even though emotionally I am all over the place. These hormones are strong. After the test is done, the consultant speaks with the manager of the clinic about my trigger. The consultant feels it is time, but the manager feels two more days may make the difference of a positive outcome. After much debate, they decide to bring me back down in two days' time, meaning two more days of injections, more money to pay. Another trip up and down the road. I cannot help feeling a little negative. I must remind myself to go with the flow more because we cannot predict how this treatment will go or guess how the schedule will be. Accept the things I cannot change.

***

Two more days, then egg retrieval, embryo fertilisation and then they will hopefully mature. It all sounds straightforward, but it is not and there will be a very anxious few days waiting.

At home, I relax and send a text to work to say I need another two days off. I should have been back tomorrow, but I am not going. In fact, I should take a week off because by the time I trigger, it will be egg collection and then hopefully transfer. Though going by the schedule, it could be the weekend before the retrieval, so I won't need time off. There I go again, trying to control what I can't. I will just go with it for the moment and maintain it as a priority and see what happens.

I get numerous texts and WhatsApp messages from Mum, Cassy and Marie wondering if everything is all right as I have been quiet. I suppose I have not been interacting on any of the social media sites as I have been busy with self-care and no drama. I imagine they know I am a little distant and they sense something is going on, though we have agreed not to say, and I feel more comfortable and a little guilty. Now I will have to cancel Tuesday yoga and meet up because I will have been in the city all day at my appointment. I decide I will ring Mum in the morning to say hi, and I will interact with others via message for now. I am so tired. Bath and bed, I think. I had a great night out on Saturday night with the girls for birthday celebrations. We had a night of great food, music and mocktails. These are non-alcoholic cocktails. I felt very pleased with myself for thinking of it and it got me out of looking suspicious for not drinking. I am usually the life and sole of the party and I still was just a sober one. I feel very blessed to have such good friendships.

I have known Cassy and Patrice from school and Marie for seven years. She was doing a course I was on and we hit it off straight away. The other two girls just clicked with her too. We all have similar senses of humour but different personalities. Before Cassy and Patrice got married, we really partied. We went on sun holidays, ski trips and murder mystery weekends. We all were lucky to gain meaningful employment straight out of college. Cassy travelled the world with her modelling career and used to take us away with her when she could. We saw some amazing sights and got an insight into the not-so-glamourous life away from the camera. We had fun though, carefree and full of enthusiasm. I wonder will all that come back in our later years when the kids are older? Mind you, by the time I have mine, the girls will be leading their second lives by that stage. Even Marie beat me to it. I believe everything happens for a reason and we might not know what it is, but you can be sure there is one.

The injections are not going so well. I've gotten them stuck in my belly, I haven't put them in far enough and I am still chewing gum which helps but it really is mind over matter. I have paced up and down the kitchen. Keith cannot cope anymore and just leaves me to it. It really is the strangest thing, the way I react to them. At this stage I will do anything. Nearly there.

Back down the road again, the conversation is light in the car. We are hoping for a good result of plenty of favourable follicles and then a date for trigger injection and egg retrieval. Keith has been struggling with the process too. He feels guilty I am going through all of this and there is nothing that he can do. Keith does not understand the whole hormonal and emotional side to this. He feels powerless and knows ultimately this is all out of our control. He talks about his feelings. Sometimes guilt, powerlessness, shame and frustration. It hasn't been easy for him and I suppose it looks like all the emphasis is on me throughout this journey. But that is only because I am the vessel, the carrier if you like. So it is important I am well physically and emotionally to give the best chance of a positive result and with us not telling anyone, he has nowhere to turn. It is very isolating, IVF. Perhaps because we have chosen not to tell anyone, and we are alone in our journey. We get the go ahead to use the trigger injection tomorrow for egg retrieval thirty-six hours after that. We are nervous and excited. At least now Keith gets to do his bit within this process, contributing his sperm for fertilisation. It is a strange feeling after the trigger, no more injections. Yippee! So potentially two more trips to the clinic. Oh, here I go again trying to work out everything I need to just chill and wait for the instructions from the consultant.

I have to fast from midnight as they use a sedative to retrieve the eggs. I have tried not to read too much into it and just go with the flow of the procedure as I might overthink it. We head back down the road again. I bring a pillow and duvet for comfort after the procedure and wear comfy clothes as advised but the nurse. Keith is nervous too, but we are not really getting into feelings today as we are both trying to be brave. When we get there, we do not even go into the waiting area. We are taken left. We have never been left before so the environment is all new to us. Everything is very clinical. I suppose this is an operation area and everything has to be to a standard. We go in and are both seated. They explain everything again, so we understand I am on the verge of hyper stimulation as my ovaries have produced a surplus amount of follicles. I change into a gown for the procedure and await the nurse. Keith and I can feel each other's nerves. The nurse calls me in, and I say goodbye to Keith. I lay on the bed for the procedure. All the relevant checks are done, and I have an injection inserted. The rest I cannot really remember. Although I was not under anaesthetic, I felt like I was out cold.

When I come to, I am awfully sick, and my blood pressure has dropped critically. Keith is horrified when he sees me, and the nurse tends to me for a while until I feel better. My ovaries have been overstimulated, and it has taken its toll on my body, so bed rest for me. We hadn't anticipated a night in hospital, but I am transferred to the local hospital for observation overnight. Keith stays in a hotel to be nearby. The next day they inform us we have seventeen embryos. They have decided not to go ahead with a straight transfer as I have overstimulated, and they will freeze the embryos. We are devastated. It has been such a rollercoaster and we both feel so upset. I shed a few tears, and the nurse tries to console me. She says it is the best option and my body will have had time to recover from the egg collection and all will be well. We try to be positive as seventeen embryos is unbelievable, and we are so lucky. This gives us a great chance of a positive outcome. We are told the clinic will ring each day and let us know how our embryos are.

It is a long journey home, and it is hard to get our heads around this journey being postponed for a month as we were in the zone if you like. And although we were finding it difficult, we were keeping our heads down and getting on with it.

I am feeling rather sorry for myself, not to mention the side effects of the overstimulation and egg retrieval procedure. There is only one thing I can do to lift my mood, and that is to spend some time with the girlies. Our relationship has been so intense, I feel Keith and I need alone time with our friends to kick start us back to ourselves again. I contact the girls via our group chat and throw the idea of some girlie time out there. Keith does the same, only his consists of beer and football. I treat myself to a new outfit and get my hair done. Well deserved, I feel. I haven't got it coloured through the process of IVF because I read somewhere the chemicals can affect the outcome. This may be just a ridiculous theory, but I am taking no chances and now is the time to do it between treatment and embryo transfer. Perhaps everything does happen for a reason. This has given Keith and I a little time to come back to ourselves and live a little again as we have been in the IVF bubble for so long. I might even enjoy a little tipple.

When I meet the girls, they are full of hugs and smiles.

'I hope you are ok,' they say.

I laugh and say, 'I'm 100% fine. Why are you all asking?'

They just look at me and agree I look great and we leave it at that. They know something is going on but have no idea what. We go to hear a local band in a hotel close to where we live. The two girls are feeling uncomfortable and do not want to go too far in case they need to pee. Patrice is in great form and she and I decide a few wee drinks will not do us any harm. Marie looks amazing and positively glowing. She is embracing her bump, she says, and is enjoying eating everything in sight. The ever body conscious Patrice tells her she will regret it after the baby is born as the weight will be hard to shift but Marie doesn't care. Cassy is different. She is watching everything she eats not for weight reasons but to ensure the baby is getting proper nutrients. She is going to pregnant yoga, swimming classes and meditation. Cassy is hoping for a hypno birth while Marie wants all the pain relief she can get. It's great to be back with the girls and be myself for a bit. I have felt so isolated. We dance a bit and chat and laugh the night away. Cassy is driving as she has the fancy jeep, and we all fit into it comfortably. At the end of the night we all get into the jeep, Patrice and I giggling as we are a little tipsy with our wine and Marie and Cassy looking at us. I'm not sure if we are annoying them or they are envious of our tipsiness. I do not feel bad as I have had a great night and a well-deserved bit of fun.

I'm feeling a little tender on the Sunday after our night out and have a lovely day relaxing in front of the fire with the dog. Even though I am feeling a little worse for wear, it a good thing as I am not feeling so intense and Keith and I are not all caught up with injections and appointments. We know that we have to wait and that we have seventeen embryos and for that we are grateful. We are just going to let ourselves heal for a while emotionally and physically.

'Back to work tomorrow.' Keith laughs.

Oh, yes. I'd forgotten about that. Oh my goodness, I better look at my emails this evening to catch up with everything. Oh, that Sunday evening feeling that Monday morning is not too far away. I love my job very much and I have worked hard to build my career, but it is funny how when you take some time off how you feel going back. I put it aside for a while and lie up with Keith in front of the fire and just enjoy some *us* time. Yummy food made by Keith, and some silly Sunday evening television and all feels well with the world.

***

Monday morning, blah. I drag myself out of bed feeling both happy and sad. Happy for normality, of just getting up and going to work without any injections. I am still feeling a little tender from the procedure, both emotionally and physically. This journey is a real rollercoaster. I have adapted a strategy of just keeping my head down and getting on with it. I am not sure what is the right thing to do, but that's what I am doing for now. I have considered counselling as it is available free from the private clinic we are having our treatment with. Purely to maintain my sanity, though I feel the worst is over with the cycle, injections and the egg retrieval and the fact we now have embryos, which is amazing. I receive a phone call to say the embryos have been growing well and will make it to blastocyst, which is the best outcome. Not all of them have made it. We have twelve now, but we are still delighted with that. They will now freeze until I get my menstrual cycle again and then the count down after that.

I need to maintain a healthy lifestyle to receive the embryos to ensure a positive outcome. I must commit to walks and proper eating to prepare my body. I just need to emotionally and mentally prepare myself. I need to ensure myself and Keith connect.

Work, work, work and no stress. My work environment usually has no stress. I come in, get an assignment and go out and investigate and write stories. At the moment we are reaching out to communities and trying to get involved in projects within the community. This is a new way of working for me in the sense I am organising events and having to do talks, lists of invites and think of workshops. While I love a challenge and embrace people; this all could not have come at a worse time. Expectations are high. On the other hand, it may be a blessing in disguise as it will distract me from watching my body clock, something that I have gotten used to over the years. It's a habit now.

It is a lovely, sunny day. I will be mindful of things and my surroundings and only say yes to things that are for my higher good. Oh, like that chocolate croissant. Now that, I feel, is good for my wellbeing now. I walk into the office and everyone is welcoming and glad to see me. When someone is off it is up to the rest of the team to help cover the call outs and bring stories to the editor.

'Ok, team meeting,' the boss says.

We all head into the boardroom. Everyone is chatting when he enters the room to discuss what needs to be covered this week and when is top priority. As the meeting goes on, I have not been allocated any of the news stories. I wonder what is going on. This is strange.

'Sam, you are in charge of the real project. I need you to develop and deliver some inspiring talks and workshops around our local community. An event. A big event. Let's say four weeks and make it big. We need to get everyone on side and not think of the newspaper in a negative light. Let's get stuck in.'

My head is spinning. BIG, he says. Community, he says and in four weeks. The most terrifying four weeks of my life and in the middle of it all I might have to go off for a while, especially if I get a call.

Ok Sam, think. Let's put this into perspective, prioritise and delegate, that's the best way. Ok team. I will pick a team.

I look around the room and slowly profile the team. I write down what reaching out to the community might look like and then I can decide who will be good to help. Women in high-profile jobs, public life, community groups and wellbeing. Yes, they can be the targets. Good, now I am on a roll. Let's get the team together and it need to be diverse and all ages involved. Eight is a good team, so eight it will be.

I put the team together and allocate roles. This is a far cry from lone working and being creative in my writing, but I love a challenge. We have speeches, workshops, marketing materials and sponsors to find. This could be a great local event and increase the function of the paper, which is always good.

Each week we will hold an event on each theme. We will locate a venue, invite guests and put ads in papers and any newsletters. This is definitely a team effort, and everyone is so committed and dedicated. It's amazing. My excitement about the project is evident and I chat about it to Mum and the girls and Keith too. They are all delighted to see me happy and excited and I am glad of the opportunity to mask my despair and anxiety beneath my happy exterior. I am really passionate about the project and can't wait to work with the team and engage with the community.

We are lucky here in the paper we have a great boss who has vision and passion and always supportive. That's because we worked together to put together a strategy, a plan of action and delegated roles. We now have a vision board and everyone in the team is committed. I love the diversity of my job and working with great people. This is a new and innovative project that will link the community and give us some coverage within wider circles. Everything happens for a reason, I suppose. Not sure about the timing, though.

The weeks fly. Work keeps me busy. I am watching my body mindfully for any wee twinge and I am being kind to myself and allowing physical and emotional recovery from the treatment. This whole process has absorbed my life, our lives. There is a strange tension between me and Keith and a knowing of anticipation that we do not want to bring into conversation for so many reasons. I'm not on my own but sometimes I feel on my own and I am sure Keith feels the same way.

***

Ok, here it goes, my time of month has come. I ring the hospital to tell them my start date and they guide me when to come in for transfer. My beautiful embryos are at blastocyst stage and have been frozen so we now have to decide how many to unfreeze with the understanding that not all of them will survive. It is amazing how attached you get to frozen embryos and the significance they hold in your life. I am grateful that it came as normal as I was worried the treatment and over stimulation might have had an impact, but thankfully no.

I will go for a nice walk this evening rain hail or shine, I feel. I text Keith to say the wheels are in motion again and we have become unstuck in our journey. I can feel the hope returning and those intense feelings that subsided for a while, return. I need to be kind to myself and positive thoughts for a positive outcome. It's just not that easy.

The morning has come. No nail polish, no earrings or perfume for the procedure. This is what we have been waiting for and are full of hope and anticipation that we are successful first time. We head back to the private clinic in through the main door and this time turn left down the corridor to the procedure unit. They ask for our identification documents to ensure the embryos are ours and consent is requested again to go ahead with the procedure. It is very surreal to be here after so many years of trying then to be told we cannot conceive unaided. To then go through the process of IVF and know today the final stage of the cycle begins. I feel my body is in a great position to receive the embryos. We have decided to have two inserted even though this can be controversial as IVF already has a high rate of twin births. We have thought about this a lot and there are a few factors that have led to us asking for two. One is my age. I am not getting any younger and we need things to happen soon. Another is financial. This has been tough on us financially and although you cannot put a price on a baby, we are not in a position to finance endless IVF treatments. We believe two gives us a better chance as two are better than one. Though it is not something that is advised, we have spoken in length to the consultant and they have agreed.

They bring us back into the room where they did the egg retrieval. This time I am fully alert. There is a nurse and a consultant. Keith is with me this time. It's a little embarrassing given what will be happening, but it is important that we are both together to see our little ones being conceived, and I need the support. Keith is beside me, and the nurse places a screen over my tummy. There is a computer screen that we can watch the procedure happening and the embryos inserted. The nurse tries to keep us at ease and explains that sometimes you can see a flash of a light when the embryo is inserted. Keith and I look at each other with excitement. I am gowned and ready to go and the consultant goes into the other room to collect the embryos in what looks like a catheter. She and the nurse verify the code on the embryos and that it matches our details, then she comes to me and begins the insertion. She uses an ultrasound on my tummy to guide her throughout and we can see this on the computer screen. It is a strange environment to be in, but I try not to think too much about it. Keith is holding my hand and I can feel his breath on my skin as he is eagerly waiting to see if there is a flash of light. We can see fully what is happening on the screen even though we are not sure what it is we are looking for. The consultant is having some difficulty locating where the embryos need to go and is moving the catheter around quite a bit. She is aware of time and is eager to position them and then a very dim white spark appears. We could just about see it.

'That's it,' she says.

I lay for a few moments before getting up and get dressed, and that is it. We say thank you, get in the car and head home on the two-hour journey back to the house. I lie on the back seat with my pillow and duvet as I have read somewhere to remain lying down after the procedure to give maximum chance of conception. It's a long journey home. I try to sleep, and Keith puts on a podcast. This is not helping, and I feel sick, so we stop, and Keith goes into a shop and buys some refreshments for us. I am not getting up. I am so aware of the implantation process I feel I must lie down to guide and protect the embryos.

When we get home, I have missed calls from Mum, work and some voice mails. I am too tired and emotional to reply, so I lie on the sofa and Keith gets me a blanket. I am feeling emotional and hopeful, full of anticipation and nesting my embryos. I am off for a few days and I intend to rest. I have read that too much lying around is not good either as I need to circulate the blood around my body. I am not sure if this is true, but I intend to give it a go. Also, eating pineapples is supposed to help with implantation so I have stockpiled these. Again, I am unsure to the accuracy of these as there is so much information out there on how to conceive, what is good for implantation, how to maintain a pregnancy and so much more. The leaflet the clinic gave me said no gym exercise for twenty-four hours or alcohol. And really that is all the advice they gave us along with suppositories and a pregnancy test which looks quite basic and a telephone number to phone with the result on a date two weeks from now.

**

The next day I rise nice and early, have pineapples for breakfast and a lovely warm shower. I feel well today, and I am trying not to think too much about the two-week wait. Which is impossible, really. I listen to my voice mails. One is Mum just ringing to see if I am still alive because she hasn't heard from me in a while. This is typical mum. The other is my boss saying I have a photo shoot this afternoon in connection with the launch of our new venture. This could not come at a worse time as I am meant to be off and resting. On the other hand, perhaps it will distract me for a few hours as my mind is constantly thinking about growing my embryos and daring to dream of my babies. I message Keith to say they've contacted me just to let him know my intentions. I might meet the girls after if they are about and that will keep me busy. I am avoiding coffee, so it might be awkward and lead to questions, but I can't keep avoiding them.

I blow-dry my hair and put some makeup on. As I am avoiding tan so no chemicals can be absorbed into my body at the moment. Trust me to be asked to do a photo shoot and no tan on. I look like a ghost. Anyhow, the things I do for my job. I head straight to the studio and meet the photographer, and he wants to take the photograph outside. Can this get any worse? I am white enough. It feels great to have other issues going on other than watching myself all the time. The photo shoot goes well, and the photographer is very interested in our project and gives me some tips and contact numbers of people he thinks might be interested in becoming involved. This has proved to be a productive few hours and excited me again about the community project. These next few weeks will be busy, and I need to look after myself.

Not all the girls are free so just Marie and I meet. She is heavily pregnant with not long to go now. She looks amazing and is truly blooming. We meet and talk about babies, relationships and swollen ankles. Poor Marie has left work early as she cannot fit into her shoes anymore. Instead of buying bigger shoes, Marie decided it was a sign to stop working and put her feet up, literally. It was lovely to hear Marie so excited about the imminent arrival of her baby and all the preparation that has happened to this point. I hear of baby kicks, morning sickness for the whole pregnancy and just that feeling of being a pregnant mum. It sounds amazing, and I am really glad we had this time together to chat. I am hopeful to soon be experiencing the same symptoms. One reason I don't want to tell anyone what I am going through is because these conversations wouldn't happen. I feel people would avoid sharing their experiences with me. I don't want sympathy; I don't want your baby and I don't compare myself to you when you are telling me about your pregnancy. I am happy waiting for my own.

It is a lovely, dry day, so we walk a little. It feels good to be out for the afternoon. I perhaps feel a little bad as Marie has shared so much with me this afternoon and I am keeping the biggest event of my life from her. Marie has really come into herself since becoming pregnant. I was so worried she was still young and has so much ahead of her that things may not turn out so well. Especially as she had considered not going through with the pregnancy. She is so glad now that she has. Marie talks of the challenges that lie ahead, maintaining her career and raising a child. She says she is up for the challenge and feels she will have plenty of support. Marie's intention is to maintain her career on her terms and be at home as much as possible. She has a great rapport with her boss, and they have already spoken about this. It is great to see employers being flexible and supporting working mums better.

After we meet, I head home, lie down and relax. I want to be kind to myself and no drama or negativity around me. Happy thoughts for a happy outcome. Two! I cannot believe I have to wait two weeks. I have to insert suppositories and they feel icky and waxy. I feel like I need a shower all the time. Too much information, I think and turn the TV on for a distraction. I need to get engrossed in a box set or a series to allow me to detach from reality for a few weeks.

***

Each day I wake I am watching my body looking for signs of early pregnancy. Every little twinge, every twitch, I am googling to see if it's a sign of early pregnancy. I am actually going to drive myself insane. This is not a new way for me as I have watched my body for years looking for signs of pregnancy and my dreams dashed every time. This time it will be different, I tell myself, filling myself with hope. I can't keep hiding away. Yet I am so distracted if I go to Mum's or meet the girls for coffee, they will all be wondering what the matter is and I cannot keep saying work. I go for a walk and come home and rest on the bed for a while and look up Netflix for a good series to start. There are a few, so I will snooze and decide later.

When I wake, I have five missed calls, two voice mails and seventeen messages. It's Marie. She has gone into labour, how exciting. I phone Keith. He sounds confused as to why I am so excited. I send Marie a message of support and then message our group chat which has been busy with the others chatting with excitement. Oh, I hope that everything goes all right and Marie is ok. It will be a long wait by the messages the girls have posted. Apparently the first child is the longest labour. It is so funny how mums know these things.

Fifteen hours later in the middle of the night the group gets a message from Marie, a picture of her and her beautiful baby girl. 7lb 7 and just perfect. Aw, I am so proud of you Marie, I type, and the others jump in too.

'It is the middle of the night,' Marie says laughing.

I cannot imagine any of us slept with the excitement of the baby's arrival. I cannot wait to meet baby Cartier tomorrow. Marie has no name picked as she was convinced she was having a boy.

Walking down the corridor of the hospital all the way to the maternity suite, it is a strange feeling. I am glad the girls are with me, even if Cassy is waddling like a duck.

'This place is making me nervous,' she explains. 'I can actually feel my waters breaking as I am that nervous,' she says laughing.

Patrice and I look nervously at each other, not knowing whether to take her seriously. Imagine if Cassy ended up in labour when in visiting Marie and her baby.

We walk into the ward and there sits Marie, looking fantastic on the bed, holding her little bundle of joy and so proud. We all give her a huge hug well done and rubbing the baby's head at the same time. It is wonderful to see Marie so radiant and proud. We have a million questions. How was labour? Have you any stitches? What pain relief? How long was labour? Marie laughs and answers them as though it was a breeze.

'Amazing, you are truly amazing,' I say. Cassy and Patrice look at me as if I have two heads and giggle.

'Excuse me, we have all done this before and you didn't think we were amazing,' they say.

I blush with embarrassment and say, 'Yes I did. I just didn't say.'

There is an awkward silence, as though the girls realise now I am the only one without a child. This is exactly why I will not be telling anyone my secret. Even now in the two-week wait when I really need someone to talk to and reassure me. I hold baby Kimie. She is beautiful, the most beautiful thing I have ever seen. I am nervous as she seems so small and delicate. The girls find my nervousness funny and joke about it. The baby cries, so I hand her back to her mama. Imagine, Marie is a mother. Goodness, I hadn't thought of that before. I have been so wrapped up in my own stuff; I hadn't taken in that Marie is now a mama. As silly as that sounds as she has been pregnant for a whole nine months. I just went with it and now it has hit me. How wonderful.

When I arrive home, Keith is there making dinner. Yum, yum. He greets me with a big hug.

'How are you?' he asks.

'I am fine,' I reply. 'Is all ok with you?

Keith admits he thought it may upset me going to the hospital and seeing a newborn baby, especially when we are going through our two-week wait. I explain. 'No, not at all. I want our baby. I never look at other babies thinking I want that baby and anyway, our little embryos are cooking away inside my tummy. I am so sure it has worked. Imagine the three of us all having babies within a year of each other. How exciting would that be?'

Time is getting so close for me to test. I am so tempted to do it early but speak with Keith and he keeps me grounded. I go back to work. There is so much to do. The project is doing really well. There are a few fundraisers and information sessions this week coming, so it will go really fast and then I can test. I just hope I do not overdo it.

The group chat is buzzing tonight with photos from earlier and the beautiful baby Kimie. She really is beautiful, and Marie is a natural already. She seemed so strong and in tune with Kimie. It really is an amazing bond, and beautiful to watch.

***

There is so much information online about IVF or ICSI, the procedure we had. This is when they insert the embryo directly into my uterus. This was the preferred option of our consultant. The online forums I find particularly useful from people who have gone through this process. As I am not telling anyone else, I have nothing else at the moment. There are other women posting about their two-week wait. We are all supporting each other and keep our spirits up whilst we are all well aware there can only be two outcomes to this, a positive or negative result, one blue line or two. Some people speak of their previous experiences, good and bad, and there are lots of tips and suggestions on how to increase your chances of a successful cycle. It's hard to process, but I just do my own thing. I enjoy the support and chat of the online forum.

***

One day to go. One day to go. I must fight off the urge to test it is two weeks for a reason. Though online, some people have done it earlier and got a positive result. I need to keep busy. I am definitely feeling twinges and little flutters, and I am excited and nervous to take the test. It can go one way or the other. It is either going to be life changing or soul destroying. Keith is aware tomorrow is the day and just gives loving glances. We do not really talk about it too much as it is so raw for us. I will go for a walk. I do not want to call anyone as they will notice I am distant and wonder what is going on. I am normally such a people person and enjoy being with others, but just at the moment it is too much.

I will go to town and get something nice for dinner. Keith will be surprised, and we can lie up this evening and imagine our positive result tomorrow. Two blue lines will be amazing and a new chapter of our lives. I smile from ear to ear even at the thought of it. I want to light the fire, but I won't as I do not want to be lifting any heavy objects as it causes harm. I suppose I should be treating myself as if I am pregnant until I know otherwise.

When Keith comes home from work, he looks like he has the weight of the world on his shoulders. I suppose when we are going through all of this it is easy to forget his feelings because the emphasis is on the female. It needs to be because it is physically and emotionally so hard on the woman. I feel I should be supporting Keith as well because it is a long, drawn-out process. I know I have not been myself for a long while now and that is because this whole process has taken so much out of me. It is hard to talk about it as it is so raw, and we are both anticipating the outcome and so hopeful of our two blue lines.

I have dinner ready and smile and give Keith a hug and a kiss. That is the best that I can do. Keith knows this and appreciates the sentiment. We both enjoy our dinner and go for a walk. My phone has been buzzing all day, but I cannot connect with anyone as I am so preoccupied with tomorrow's results.

I have a shower and some lovely scented candles to relax myself and hope I sleep. I can really feel the tension and the nerves are definitely there for tomorrow morning. They say to use first urine as it is the strongest and for the best result. Tomorrow is the day we find out if all those tests and trips to the city and not to mention the injections and hormones have worked. We dare to dream and feel the delight in becoming parents after waiting for so long. It is hard not to get your hopes up, especially when the process has taken years to get to this point. I just have a feeling it has definitely worked, and we are one of the lucky ones who managed to be successful first time. I can definitely feel something is happening.

This is it! This is it! I unwrap the test from the paper cover. I read the instructions again and again to make sure I know what to do. It is 6am I can't wait any longer. Keith is awake too. I think he would come in and watch me pee on the stick if he could.

I pee on the stick and wait...

One blue line. My heart sinks. Keith looks at me to react and I can't. I am numb. One blue line.

I cannot speak. I need to cry and cry, but the tears won't come. Still sitting on the bathroom floor, Keith gives me a hug, and we hold each other. I swear he can feel my pain. He is shaking too. We get up, move to the bedroom and just lie there holding each other, our dreams dashed. An empty feeling comes over me. I fall asleep with Keith holding me. I need to feel. Who would have thought the power of one blue line could have? My stomach is wrenching.

When I wake the sun has come out. It is shining into my room. I have a blanket over me, and Keith is downstairs, I think, as he is not here, and I can hear some rattling about downstairs. I sit up on the bed. It is now 11.20am. Keith should be at work. I am not sure I can face the day. It's too hard. Is that it? Is that really it? No baby after all of that. Surely if they implanted the embryos into me, they should grow. They have to grow. Why wouldn't they? All these questions are going around in my head. I really thought it worked. I was feeling twinges and niggles, and my tummy felt funny. I cannot believe it.

Keith comes up. He has made me some brunch. I ask him why he is not at work and he says he has booked the day off. He thought we would either be celebrating or devastated, so either way he wanted to be here. I start to cry, and Keith puts the tray down and comes and sits beside me on the bed. He knows I am so upset and realises I really thought it worked. He holds me tight, trying to squeeze my pain away.

'How can this be?' I ask?

Keith tries to console me by saying it is all right. We can try again. All is not lost. But that is not what I want to hear. I wanted it to work this time. I wanted the embryos to grow inside me and for us to be a family. I am not sure I can go through the whole process again. It really took its toll on me emotionally and physically and I do not think we can survive. I just cry. I lie back down on the bed again and decide I am not facing the day and I am not ringing the clinic with my result either. I cannot bear to say the words. Empty is how I am feeling right now, and I do not know how to deal with it. I lie upstairs and Keith goes back down. This is a very isolating journey.

I cry tears and tears. How did it not work? I cannot understand. Surely if the embryos were put in the place they need to be, they'd grow, and I would be pregnant. Where did they go? I have no sign of anything. If anything, I have been getting twinges and feelings of pregnancy. It must still be in there. Perhaps I tested early. I have often heard of this and the test didn't show pregnant until weeks later. That's it. I will wait. All is not lost. I will get up, shower, put my face on and take the dog for a walk. I need to blow away the tears.

I go downstairs after my shower and Keith looks very surprised to see me. He looks upset. His hopes have just been dashed as much as mine. I rub his shoulder and tell him it will be all right. I explain my new logic and I'm not sure if he is horrified or in agreement. We decide to go for lunch and a walk. I will still eat sensibly, just in case. Keith is very quiet during our walk and doesn't say much. I am mindfully trying to take in our surroundings. The wind is refreshing, and it is giving me hope, hope for our future and the baby we so desperately want. I really need to reengage with family and friends, and I had promised myself after the two-week wait I would, but it is more complicated now. Marie must feel I have abandoned her and her new baby, so I must set myself a target to visit. I am sure that it is not that easy being a first-time mum. Patrice and Cassy are so busy, I imagine they haven't noticed much, and we are keeping in touch via the group chat.

Keith interrupts my trail of thought and asks me when I will phone the clinic to tell them the result. He fears if I do not phone, they will start phoning me. I explain I am not ready to yet as that would make it seem real and as if there is no hope. Keith looks at me in a concerned manner and I just smile back at him saying, 'A woman knows her own body and I do not believe it is over yet.' We continue to walk in silence.

***

I set my alarm that night as I am back to work tomorrow. I am looking forward to it and not. I am so distracted with what is going on I feel people will notice and yet I need the distraction of work. Our community workshops are about to be launched, and it is a very exciting time to be at the newspaper. We are very lucky to have such support from higher management and their commitment to improve wellbeing is commendable.

I get up as usual, shower, dress and head down for breakfast. Keith is busy packing lunch to head out the door. We have a brief chat about our day ahead and he heads on, leaving me with a kiss, of course.

Work is a great place to be. Even in the intense environment of targets and deadlines, we still manage well as a team. Tuesday is a heavy day getting everything out to print, ensuring we are on the pulse and up to date with local events. People's stories are amazing, and this is why I first entered the world of journalism. My curiosity for life and love of people. I have a good morning and phone Cassy about lunch. Cassy is both surprised and delighted to hear from me and automatically assumes I have news. I can only assume it was baby news that she was looking for. I don't think people realise how hard that question is or upsetting.

I meet with the team, and we draw up a timetable for our events and workshops. Everyone is both nervous and excited. This is a new venture for us, and we do not know how we will be received in the community. The newspaper has done a great piece of coverage with a good response on social media, which is encouraging. I am enjoying this piece of work as it is not too strenuous, yet it fills my days and occupies my mind.

***

Marie looks fantastic, and motherhood really suits her. She effortlessly tends to baby Kimie. She is excited to see me and tells me all her plans for the baby's christening and her modern take on the event. I cannot believe how big a baby can grow in one week and I am fascinated how a mother's instinct can kick in. We stay in the house because Marie does not want to take Kimie out in the cold. This suits me just fine. I am happy chatting and gushing over the baby. I've never seen so much pink. I get all the gory details of the birth and look at how proud Marie is of herself. Super woman springs to mind. How fantastic it is when nature does its job. The miracle of life is quite something, and the process of new life is amazing.

I head home feeling happy and sad. What a lovely afternoon I had with one of my closest friends and her new baby. I feel so proud and delighted for Marie. I feel a little sad for me, holding out hope the 20th pregnancy test was wrong. That somehow, I am l pregnant and against all odds. Keith is right. I need to phone the clinic with my results.

I phone the clinic and listen to the sympathetic nurse on the end of the phone. She tells me I may not menstruate straight away as I was stuck on the notion I must be pregnant if I have not had my period, but this is not the case. The nurse explains that when I am ready, I should phone for an appointment to come back down to discuss the next step and our options. After all, we still have some grade A embryos left and they can be kept in storage. I don't even consider this at this time and just say my goodbyes and hang up. I text Keith to say I have made the call, and he appears glad of the closure.

Life goes on. I cannot just get on with things. This is constantly on my mind, so many questions. Why did it not work? Why is Keith not like me? I really believed it would happen straight away.

A holiday! That's it. We need to go on a holiday. I need to detach, get past the pain and have something to look forward to. Oh, I wonder if I would get time off work? Can we afford it? This IVF journey has proven expensive and any money we have left is for another round should we decided to try again. Oh, my goodness, I can't even think about it. I'm still grieving the failed attempt. That's it. I'm grieving. That's how I feel. Even though there was no baby, I'm still grieving the failed attempt from the process. Oh, I need to talk to someone. This is a lot tougher than I thought it would be. There is counselling support with the private clinic. I phone the number and arrange an appointment. Unfortunately, it is in the same area the clinic is and there is no one else closer. This is one of the many disadvantages to living so rural. I now must decide if this is a viable option as it will take a whole day to attend one appointment. Perhaps they can do evenings. I will wait until they contact me and ask. Nothing is ever simple, and I am finding it hard not to feel overwhelmed. This is a new feeling for me and not one I am used to have to deal with or consider. I have to relax and slow down my breathing and thoughts.

Later that evening, I decide to give meditation a go again with Keith. It worked before. Perhaps it will work again. I find it hard to slow my thoughts, stop tears flowing from my eyes and maintain some normality. I really felt strong and capable before the negative result. I felt like I could conquer the world juggling a job, a marriage and the biggest secret of my life. I discuss with Keith a holiday and we agree on a weekend away and save our money for any future procedures we may need.

Ok, meditation it is. There is too much going on. We bring the White Tara mantra to our meditation and visualise a baby and ask for help. Keith has researched this so much. I admire his belief. It may make a difference. I suppose we all need hope and belief that something bigger than us can help. I go online that evening and book a hotel not too far away. It has a pool and a spa, and we can avail of these facilities whilst there. It's good to get away somewhere that is not work related or treatment related. And it takes back some control and a sense of making our own decisions and not being dictated to by a cycle of IVF.

***

The next day I head to work as normal. Looking forward to a weekend away, I keep my head down and continue supporting the team with the new project. I ensure we have everything covered and everyone is up to speed with the rotas and agenda of the work we'll do within the community.

Every team is different and are microcosms of families. It's funny to watch and to relate to. The team at the newspaper are no different and I have to ensure we are flawless in our approach to reach out and yet be relatable. We have all the marketing material ready and I must say it looks very impressive. The team have excelled themselves. This is new territory for us all the excitement is building and so far, we have been well received. People's perception of journalists can be varied. Some embrace us and some avoid us. It depends on their experiences with the press. We need to accept the good with the bad and neither should affect us, neither praise nor negativity.

We have the timetable set and all guest speakers confirmed. This will be a great project, and everyone needs to be committed, including myself. Community wellbeing is so important and in our little community we have had our fair share of tragedy and loss. Being a journalist, I see this first-hand. The team and I feel we can get the community together to make a difference, getting local heroes and super stars to speak about their wellbeing and how different things can impact. That it's important to keep it local and relatable to us here in the community. Some organisations are resistant to the project and some embrace it. People dislike change or controversy, and our intention is not to upset anyone. We are looking to raise awareness and support those in need or try to prevent need and educate on promoting wellbeing. Everyone is dedicated to this and have been innovative in their approach and included many people within their circle to develop the workshops and materials. I am looking forward to the launch next week.

Keith is worried I may have taken on too much. The last thing I would want Keith to think is that I would jeopardise our chances of having a baby for my work. It's a welcome distraction right now and sure it's nothing physical and so long as I ensure time off and self-care, all will be well.

I decide it's time to face Mum, so I call to say hello. She knows something is going on. Goodness only knows what she is filling in the blanks with. I bring biscuits. Dad is there when I arrive. This is good as it means there will be only chit chat and Mum never gets into a deep conversation when Dad is about. We discuss the usual things, the world, the rest of the family and I chat endlessly about work, deciding to use this excuse why I have not been about in a long time. Mum rightly points out the missed calls and texts I did not reply to. I have no excuse for this and the look on my face displays guilt. I'm certain Mum knows this. I offer to bring Mum shopping at the weekend to get her out of the house. I do this hesitantly as I fear she will pry, but I have always done this, so I need to maintain it. It's not Mum's fault I am going through this and I really don't want to say. I am acting different. I know this, and it is because I am different. I have been through so much and now the feeling of loss has engulfed me.

Chapter 7

The Next Phase

Even when you are busy and thinking of other things, this feeling you have just won't go away. It's as if it is sitting on your shoulder or in the pit of your stomach. Even when you are not consciously thinking about having a baby you are. I try to explain this to the allocated counsellor. I really need to shake the failed attempt off as when Keith and I went for our weekend break we agreed to give it another try. We spoke about a non-medicated cycle this time as it was the intensity of the injections we feel affected us as a couple and individually. A non-medicated cycle means no injections and you follow the cycle of your body. You contact the clinic on day one of your cycle and then monitor your ovaries and then implantation on the day they feel you are most favourable to take the embryos. They will now need to thaw some of our embryos, and we need to hope for the best they survive the thaw. We are only at the discussion stage and I need to phone the clinic to arrange an appointment to speak with the consultant yet. That is why I am here trying to get my head around the first cycle and accept it before I move on to another one. It's a strange thing, infertility. It's a very isolating experience to go through and the rollercoaster ride and heartache no one would understand unless you go through it. And it's quite a taboo subject. Look at me. I won't even tell anyone. This is for many reasons but still, like mental health, there is a stigma to it and a risk of being judged.

The counsellor is a pleasant woman. She wants Keith to come next time. I'm not sure how he will feel about that. I look up support groups in the area as I feel I need someone to talk to. Perhaps complete strangers are the best people to talk to and ones who have been or are going through a similar experience. The groups are a bit far away, but everything is from where I live. I search endlessly online for information and forums just to equip myself for round two and to not feel as isolated.

On the way home, I call in to see Patrice. I just need some female company and a friendly face and a cup of tea. This is my way of self- care. I feel so tender after the counselling session and I didn't feel like we spoke a lot about anything except my journey, which I felt I was very black and white about. It's dark when I arrive at Patrice's house. The kids are in bed, and she is in the kitchen making the tea. She was expecting me as I had phoned beforehand. I am glad to see her and make some excuses why I have not been in touch much lately and I've neglected our regular coffee and cake catchups. I say I have been so busy with work and explain the new project I am involved in. I invite Patrice to come with me to some of the events. They are during school time, so it should suit. Patrice seems interested and says she will come. She looks across the table at me and smiles, to which I burst out crying. This has just come out of nowhere. Patrice jumps up to get me a tissue and asks me what is wrong. I cannot hold it in any longer and I explain what I have been going through and how I am feeling. The tears just keep coming and the pain is so real and raw, I am not sure what I feel or what is happening. I feel a release with the tears and the words. My secret is not a secret anymore and now

I will have someone to confide in and help me through it. Just then, Patrice's phone rings.

I am so distraught. I didn't think she would answer the phone as I had said what a big deal it was for me to share this and how I had not told anyone else. But Patrice does answer the phone and chats calmly to the lady on the other side as I am sitting full of tears and so inconsolable, I could not speak. Patrice chats for another minute or so, hangs up the call and offers me another tissue.

She says, 'I'm calling over to see Jane. Do you want to come?'

I look at her in disbelief. I just confided my biggest secret ever and needed support, and Patrice has completely dismissed me in my time of need. Perhaps I've asked too much. Maybe I'm being silly. Why would anyone support me? But then again, why not? Is that not what friends are supposed to do. It was such a big deal for me to tell anyone, and I felt I'd explained that to Patrice, that she would have understood. Instead, I am responded to with an invite to a girl across the park for a bit of meaningless gossip and a chit chat. I am lost for words. I know everyone has their own things going on, but my goodness this hurt. Driving home, I am still crying. I feel sad, hurt and stupid for telling my secret and looking for support. This has just re-affirmed I need to tell no one and just hope Patrice is true to her word and tells no one. Although given her response to my crisis, I am not counting on that.

When I get home, Keith is there. He can clearly see I was crying. He knew I was calling in to Patrice's and cannot understand why I am upset. Keith sits me down and asks if I am all right. I start to cry again and tell him all about my day with the counsellor, what it brought up for me, and that she wants us both to attend a session. As I suspected Keith is not keen, but I am not too worried about that at the moment. I then tell him about my visit with Patrice and what happened. He just held me close and kissed my head. Keith doesn't say very much. I am not sure what his thoughts are. I cannot process how I am feeling about this evening, never mind trying to work out what Keith is thinking. I cannot even eat. I just run a lovely bath and lie and soak until my hands wrinkle.

Oh, what a rollercoaster! I don't know what I am feeling, whether I am coming or going. I know I have a lot to do at work and some big decisions to make regarding taking another leap of faith on our IVF journey. Perhaps I am oversensitive, but there and then in my bathroom I decide that will never happen to me again. This is my journey along with Keith's. I need to protect myself and us from any emotional distress, so I will keep myself to myself and get on with it. Sad, but it's true. This is the way it has to be. I should never have said anything, and I hope Keith is not annoyed. I go downstairs feeling much better having taken back my power and made my decision. I am much happier. People are not used to me being the vulnerable one. They do not like it or expect it, which is unfortunate for me in my time of need, but nothing that will keep me down for long.

Mmm, hot chocolate. Keith knows me too well. If I am not eating, I will never refuse a hot chocolate and some nice biscuits. That will get me every time. Now I am safe at home all snug with my nightgown on, fire lit, Harry lying up beside me and Keith preparing lunch for tomorrow. Pure bliss at the end of an awful day.

***

Up for work and back to it. I have no time to mull over yesterday. I have decided to put it behind me. I have too much to think about. Our project launches this week and I have some last-minute details to tie up. I need Excel sheets, emails and courtesy phone calls made to every business and organisation attending. If everything goes to plan, this will be amazing, so I need to make sure everything is flowing well, and the team are communication with each other. Our marketing material arrives, and this excites us. It re-energises the team, not that we needed it. What a great team we are. People from all departments coming together for a common good. I am so glad to be part of this. I do a lot of travelling with my job and networking and dealing with the public, so this project is a great opportunity to use all my skills. I am still nervous though. Nervous for the success of the project to make a difference and get people to talk about wellbeing.

My boss comes down today to chat. He is usually pleasant and easy to work with, but today he has a different tone. Today the nerves are beginning to show, and he is argumentative and bossy. That might sound strange calling a boss bossy, but he is not usually like that. He is fussing about things regarding the project that are irrelevant and throwing words around aimed to hurt. I am feeling vulnerable enough at the moment and find it hard to take. I feel like people can pick up on my energy and know that I am a little tender, and they decide to make me feel even worse. I'm not sure why this is happening, but I can feel it. Perhaps I am giving hints away, or I am not functioning as I normally do. All I know is people are picking up on it and it is affecting our interactions. I'm not sure if that is even a thing. I know that it has happened to me on several situations now and I am not my usual feisty self. It seems to give people the impression they can be rude or nasty to me.

What to do? What to do? Should we go again? I cannot get the embryos out of my head. They are our embryos, the start of life, our babies, so it's a no brainer to me. My mind would not let me leave them. I have researched non-medical approach and with me being so regular; I feel we have a high chance of success this time. Perhaps all the medical intervention and over stimulation affected our success the last time. Gosh, even the fact I can process that means I am recovering from our negative cycle. The counselling must be working. Pity I could not get Keith to go. I feel it has really helped me. I never thought I would be going for counselling support and definitely for fertility support. It has taught me to have an open mind more and not be so black and white about things.

I still feel as though I need to protect myself and be guarded if I am giving out signals of vulnerability and people are picking up on this. I need to be guarded, and I feel that is ok.

At work I am attending an awards ceremony with colleagues from other regions. I am usually chatty and sociable, though not so much these days, especially since the impact of a cycle. I sit at a table towards the back of the room. There are only two people sitting at the opposite side of the table initially, so I feel happy to be there. It does not take long for more to join us. The table fills quickly, some directors of the company and some of my colleagues alike. Neill sits down.

'Hi Sam. How are you? I haven't seen you in ages,' he says.

I reply with a smile, and we chat for a while. We talk about work, and how busy it is. He is keen to hear more about our new project and admits he would love to be part of it and how it was a pity he was so far away. I giggle, feeling proud our little space is the first to implement the new project and reach out to the community. Neill asks how Keith is, and I tell him he is doing well. Neill then asks the dreaded question.

'Any sign of starting a family yet?'

I do not know why people ask me that all the time, I look down for a second and reply, 'Gosh no. I'm too busy with work at the moment. Give us time.' I try to laugh it off. 'What about you?' I ask. 'No sign of the pitter patter of little feet either?'

Neill, who is sitting right beside me, shakes his head.

'No, unfortunately. It's not for us. We have tried for many years with no success. We had four cycles of IVF that were unsuccessful, and it nearly drove us apart. It was so tough on Sandra. We just had to be honest with each other and stop trying.'

I looked at Neill and apologised for asking and he told me not to be silly, that they have accepted it now and enjoy the life they have. He also said he is just honest about it now when people ask. He does not hide the fact. I admired his honesty though I am not in that place yet but hope to be some day. I commented, 'Why do people always ask that question anyway? I usually don't, but in response to your question I thought it was ok. He laughed at my apology and related to exactly where I was coming from. He spoke about Sandra's journey and her self-care and how important it was to the process. Neill also spoke of his feeling of helplessness in the physical side of the cycle being so demanding on Sandra. I could really relate to his words. I was glad I sat where I was as even though my intention was to fade into the background, I received information I really needed to hear. Although Neill was never successful, they tried until they were exhausted, and I am not there yet, although one cycle had really taken its toll. I was sitting exactly where I was meant to at exactly the right time. I did feel a little guilty for keeping my secret and not confiding in Neill, but after all, he choose to be so open and I just couldn't. Especially after what had happened with Patrice and any how I was at work. I comforted myself with that thought.

***

I have a fresh new perspective and a little hope regained. I cannot wait to tell Keith about chatting to Neill today. It was so good to hear from someone else and even though I did not reciprocate; I got so much out of our conversation. Neill will probably never know. I completely zoned out about the awards. I was engulfed in the conversation with Neill and my thought of processing his journey. I need to jump back to work mode. It is amazing what people can achieve. Today's diversity awards have shown me that. I go back to the office to finish editing my piece I wrote yesterday; deadlines are a hard thing to follow when you are distracted and trying to keep a secret, hide your despair and deal with hormones. Yes, my cycle is back with a vengeance, and I am really feeling it. I am glad though as it also gave me closure.

I go uptown after work and browse. It's only now I also realise I lost myself a little as I seem to be able to see more things up the town and notice new things I hadn't for a while. I decide to be kind to myself and get my nails done in a new nail bar that takes non appointments. How cosmopolitan. I think these services do not usually come here. I go to the bakery and pick up some treats for the evening. When Keith gets home, I excitedly tell him about my conversation with Neill today. Keith is a little confused why I am excited as their treatment did not work, but that was not what I gained from the conversation. I got hope and courage to go again and try for my baby that I so want. I explained I just needed time, time to heal and process the loss. I really feel we are not the only ones going through this and it is more common than we realise, and we need to try. Keith agrees and we decide to make the call to the clinic tomorrow for our follow up appointment to discuss options and have any questions answered we may have.

We relax that evening, get a takeout, chill, and I start to believe again.

***

The next day I get up as usual and get ready for work. It is less than a week for the launch and I have plenty to do, but all that I can think of is making the phone call for another appointment. This is it, you see. Once I start the journey; it takes over even when I do not realise it. I am more aware this time and will try not to let it happen as much. I leave the house and head for the office. I plan to phone in the car. I need to leave now to miss the traffic going into town. Traffic is slow as always, so I turn the radio on to pass the time. After circling the office for what seemed an eternity, I finally get a space, park, and dial the number for the clinic. I'm a little nervous, but that's ok I feel. A pleasant lady answers the phone. I explain the situation and give my details. Everything comes rushing back to me and I remember my feelings throughout the process. I breathe in a deep breath and allow myself to recover from the feeling.

'Ok, so we have an appointment available next week to speak with a consultant,' she says.

Ahh next week, I think to myself, *that's the launch I can't really do it. I do not want to stress myself out.*

'Oh gosh, 'I reply, 'I'm sorry. Next week doesn't suit me.' I feel guilty for not taking the first appointment available as it seems I am not keen, but that is not the case. It's just too much. This is something I have learned. I need to know when to say no. A week or two will not make any difference, our beautiful embryos are still there waiting and frozen for us.

I arrange the next appointment and feel satisfied I have taken back a little control and I feel hope rushing back in along with fear. I message Keith to tell him when the appointment is and now, I will move on and concentrate on work. I am really excited about our work project. It is different to what we are used to. I know it will be busy as I still have to do my main job alongside this, but the team are great, and the enthusiasm is infectious. We really feel passionate about engaging with the community and promoting change.

The launch will be one of its kind. We've sent invitations out, replies are now in. The team have workshops prepared, guest speakers have confirmed, and we are awaiting the last bit of marketing materials. I enjoy the buzz of a committed team with all the same enthusiasm for what we are trying to achieve. Reaching out to the local community to promote positive wellbeing and connections is something we all feel passionate about.

In the middle of all of this I have a little family who are sitting back watching me keeping busy. I feel I am always doing something while they have no clue of what I am going through. I feel slightly deceitful, but it is the only way we can cope. I am sure they know something is amiss but never in their wildest thoughts would they know it was IVF and that there was an issue at all. They think I'm a career girl and always doing something interesting. Yet in reality I yearn for the quiet life with my baby, happily letting the fast-paced career lifestyle take a back seat.

The launch day has come. The excitement and nerves are plain to be seen. Everything has been organised and if it all falls into place, the event will be very successful. We gather for a debrief and the energy is high, a real positive vibe. It is really encouraging to work with so many great people who have the same passion and vision to connect with the community and become involved. Our work can be controversial at times depending on what is happening and what job we are assigned to do. Getting involved with the community is why I got into journalism in the first place and getting the truth for people.

The launch went amazingly well. The rooms were full. We received plenty of feedback and some bookings for future engagements and workshops. I am so glad the project has launched and has received a positive response, and going forward, it will grow.

***

Ok, so here we go back down the road again. My stomach is in triple knots. My head is spinning with lots of questions. Why did it not work? Is it my fault? What can I do to make it work next time? Keith is not really saying much, and that is ok, I understand. It is a long journey to the clinic emotionally and in miles. I cannot explain the feeling the journey stirs up. I am feeling strong and brave though so I will keep an open mind. We have touched on the subject of where is our end point and neither of us are there yet, so moving forward is the only way.

We reach the clinic; an all too familiar sight and we enter and sign ourselves in at the desk and take our place in the waiting room. Nothing has changed. Keith goes straight for the coffee machine as always and I lift the magazines and have a read through. People come and go. We all give each other a nod as we enter and leave, everyone knowing why each one is there, and the hopeful anticipation is evident. As they guide us down the corridor, we chat loosely with the nurse and she explains the doctor will be with us in a moment. I have all my notes with me and highlighted any points I need clarity on and questions I have. When the doctor comes in, he sits down and is very matter of fact.

He says, 'Right then, are we going again?'

I am taken aback by his promptness and say, 'No, we need to discuss the last cycle and why it was unsuccessful.'

He looks at our notes on his computer screen and says, 'Really, I have no answers. It is more common that it does not work the first time.'

I ask if there is anything that we could have done, and he explains, no, that all went according to procedure. He looked again at our notes and referenced how many grade A embryos we have left and said we should try again. I said I felt the over stimulation affected the success and played a factor. The consultant feels that we are lucky we have such good grade embryos and we should go again. I explain the trauma I felt with all the injections and the pressure of the whole cycle. We talk for some time about treatment and the process, and Keith and I raise the potential for a non-medical cycle. The doctor is not as keen for non-medical as it relies heavily on my cycle pattern. I assure him my cycle is regular, and I am confident I can easily track it.

So, what I need to do is register at the clinic for a non-medical cycle and phone in when my period comes. Then they will call me down then to track my ovulation and work out a timetable on that. A non-medicated cycle is not injection free and we will still have to attend regular appointments, but it means I am letting my cycle occur naturally. I feel much happier with this decision. It feels right. I am confident my body will accept the embryo with limited intervention and less stress on Keith and I. So, we make an appointment and payment for our new cycle. It costs less than a medicated cycle, but you still have to pay for some meds and the procedures. Keith is feeling calmer there won't be a stream of medication in our fridge or the dreaded few weeks of me injecting myself and feeling hormonal and anxious. The journey back down the road again is a pleasant one. We stop for some food and feel relaxed and happy in each other's company. It really takes its toll on your relationship and it is there all the time at the back of your mind. It is nice to find us for a time.

We get home and light the fire. It is not cold but there is something relaxing about it. I run a bath and soak up all the information received today. This could all happen quickly as we do not need to wait for anything except for my cycle to be regular and contact the clinic. Statistically, there is not much of a difference in success rates, so I am confident.

***

Up and back at it tomorrow and I look forward to catching up with the girls this week. It has been ages and this time it is really is because work has been so busy. I am still buzzing from the launch. Our diary is now full of events for engaging with the community, which has been a success.

I meet with the girls, all except Patrice as she declined the WhatsApp invite. The others are happy to see me. We meet at our usual spot, this time a little earlier and with little babies on toe. They are so cute. How things have changed from cocktails and a' la carte menus. It is now energetic, and food is going everywhere. I enjoy the fun and find myself repeatedly telling the girls not to worry and to stop apologising. I love it. Kids are so cute and lively. They keep us young. We eat, drink tea and come alive with the kids. All is well. It feels so good to reconnect and having work to talk about helps keep the conversation going. The girls look tired with not much sleep being had at this stage but all worth it. Life just takes over and after having children, time is so precious and can go by so quickly.

Chapter 8

Second chance

Here we go. Cycle has been tracked, trigger has been dated and all set to go. My beautiful cousin Isla, whom I am so close to, has just started uni. I feel so sad I could not be there with her when she moved. This is something we talked about for so long. I feel bad to have let her down on this occasion. This is just one of many. I have to stay here and track my ovulation and wait for the trigger. Poor Isla has rung to say she is so sick with Freshers Flu, they call it. She sounds so poorly; her friends are looking after her, but I just want to jump on a plane and look after her. This is what I would normally do but can't because of the treatment. I feel so bad and Isla sounds so sick. Please let this be successful this time and all this will be worth it. The feelings and emotions I have endured over the last few years surely have been a rollercoaster. Everything has an impact and IVF takes over everything with no mercy. I try to change my thinking and try self-care to ease the impact, but it never seems to work. I still feel guilty, anxious, secretive and every other emotion under the sun regularly on a daily basis. Yet the yearning will not go away and everything will be all right if we could just get pregnant and have a healthy baby or babies. My life would be complete.

Back down the road again, the long road to the clinic. Lots of thoughts going through my head between conversation and songs on the radio. Hoping this will all be worth it and trying to stay positive. We arrive at the clinic, and this time it is straight in and turn to the left. It's all too familiar and I try to destroy any negative thoughts or fear from my mind. We have decided to stay in a hotel this time to give the embryo its best chance. This time it is a male consultant who will complete the procedure. The nurse is there, and they check all the details on my band and the embryos. I feel excited. I see the ultrasound machine and remember how it went the last time. Keith is with me and we both smile at each other nervously. We have put so much into this emotionally, physically and financially. I put my gown and hat on and prepare myself for the procedure. It is a strange-looking instrument and I suppose it is more uncomfortable than anything else. The doctor comes in. He is gowned and ready to go. The nurse gives him the embryo in the tube and here we go, lying on the bed, hoping for success. I watch the screen. Because of the Doppler on my stomach, I can see the tube going in and watch patiently to see it being inserted. The doctor doesn't seem confident. In fact, he takes it out and puts it back in again. Eventually he retreats. We look at him for reassurance, and he says it's in there now. We smile at each other.

The doctor says, 'How many more embryos do you have left?'

We reply, 'Six.'

'Ah, good.'

At that point, Keith and I look at each other. I can feel my heart sinking. I'm no mind reader, but those words and the lack of confidence in the procedure are telling me this has not worked. I lie for a few minutes and get up when instructed by the nurse. I get dressed, sign some forms and leave for the hotel feeling very deflated and not excited or hopeful like last time. I hadn't expected to feel like this, but something is telling me it hasn't gone according to plan. We check in and I lie on the bed and have a short nap. Keith is sitting up reading and when I come around, we chat a little and decide we need to stay positive as there is a possibility our baby could be growing in me. We need to give loving thoughts from the start and be mindful of our energy and thoughts.

So, I relax and breath and become mindful of the embryo growing and burrowing its way to achieve a positive pregnancy. I feel excited now and Keith and I cuddle and dream. We order room service and I lie with my legs elevated hoping this will help with the process. We have been here many times before when we were tracking cycles, ovulations and best ways to achieve a positive result. The years of trying and investigations it has taken even before we get to this stage, I feel grateful to be here now and have a second chance. The non-medical cycle has worked to this point. We could monitor everything and trigger when needed. I am used to all the intrusive tests and procedures now. I don't pass much remarks as the outcome will be wonderful if achieved. Never in a million years did I think I would be in this situation, something I probably took for granted. I would fall in love, get married, set my career and have kids. It is a real kick to the stomach to find out it won't be that easy and that one blue line would have some much heartache and significance in my life.

***

The next day we head for home back down the long road again. It is a sunny day and there are lots of people out and about. Sunny weather always makes you feel better and we don't get much of it here, so it is lovely when we see it. I enjoy long, rain-free days. They allow me to slow down and take it all in. My life is so busy most of the time with work, and the constant underlying issues with fertility time seems to go so quickly. I rest for a few days, just to recover emotionally. Keith goes back to work, and I am ok with this as it can be very tense. He just looks at me almost as though he is looking for a sign or a glimmer it has worked. I cannot give any hope or indication. I was so sure that it would work the last time. I am happy to throw my hands in the air this time and say I have no idea. The two-week wait or the TWW as some call it is particularly hard as you are monitoring everything and just desperately hoping all of your efforts have paid off.

I need to fill my days as this consumes every minute of the day and night. Having a conversation with Keith other than IVF is hard. We lose our relationship in this process but are aware it will not be this way for long. Some people probably get closer, each to their own. Couples are three times more likely to break up or get divorced after failed IVF. I do not want to be one of those couples. But I can identify with the highs and lows and the stressors that IVF can have on an individual's mental health and on relationships, especially when it does not work. Tensions can be high, so self-care is so important right now.

Keith has a great way of approaching this as he has many outlets. I'm private and often wear my heart on my sleeve. I find it hard not to be confiding in others and I feel you can tell by my face I am hiding something so I recluse for self-preservation. This really does not suit my personality as I can be outgoing.

Lots of pineapple, good food and no alcohol, no stretching or stress for the next few weeks. I really want to give this the best I can as I do not know if we can go through this all again for so many reasons. I will go back to work and keep my head down and not let any stress affect me. I will try not to show I'm feeling vulnerable at the moment as I really do feel people pick up on it and attack.

Keith is keeping himself busy. I am trying, but my every thought is watching my body, waiting for a sign.

And just like that... our dreams and hopes for a future of three are dashed. One blue line. A complete negative. No baby. It hasn't worked. We knew in the bottom of our hearts it hadn't worked based on the reaction of the doctor and the questions he was asking about how many embryos we had left. Still, that gut-wrenching feeling comes back, the pain of a negative result no easier than the last time. Even though I definitely pulled back and did not allow myself to go back to that place, it still hurts. It hurts a lot.

There are no words. Loss, grief, sadness, pain are words that I can use to describe the feeling. I just want to crawl into bed and not get out. This is so hard, so unfair. Why us?

***

For the next few days I will choose self-care. This is a word often thrown around and potentially not utilised enough, but I need it now I need to be kind and let myself heal. I need not to think of Keith or work or anyone else, just me for now, the vessel who so wants to carry a new life and bring a child into the world. I refuse to torment myself on what I should have done or could have done. I don't think I can do this again.

Long walks and girlie chats. This is why I am glad that no one knows what I have been through. No pity, no shame or endless conversations around why it didn't work, to be cheerful, it will happen next time.

We went for coffee. Oh, how I have missed this. We have change venue from our lovely cake and coffee in the evening to a children's play centre coffee shop with screaming children in the background. The idea is to let the children exhaust themselves ready for bed when they get home. The girls look great. Me on the other hand, I look tired exhausted from the emotional rollercoaster. I pass it off as work deadlines when Marie comments on my appearance.

'Is everything all right with Keith?' is the next question.

'Yes,' I say, 'of course.'

Cassy is still having doubts about the au pair. I'm not sure why as Cassy is a beautiful lady with a high-end modelling career. Although she doesn't do as much modelling anymore, she is a powerhouse of the industry and has her own fashion brand. Her kids adore her and her husband even more so. We spend the next half an hour telling her so. Oh, it's so good to be talking chit chat with the girls, the kids have gotten so big and life is treating them well. Marie is the biggest shock. She has taken to motherhood so well and is just enjoying her time being a mum and building a career and life around it. Patrice and I decided life is too short to hold grudges. To be honest, I do not have the emotional energy to keep up an argument, so I decide to chat even though our relationship is fractured during our meet up. Patrice has decided to go back to learning and gain some qualifications. We all find it so funny that our coffee link up is now not so cosmopolitan and more mummy. I enjoy it all the same. I don't feel envious, just a little sad that my little one is just not going to come that easy, if they come at all.

By now, I am just getting on with life. The mental, emotional and financial strain of two failed cycles have taken their toll and we are getting on with things. Back to work, going for walks, nights out and fitting in yoga class. Yoga is good for me. Keith should come too, but he doesn't see the benefits. My tummy still looks like a pincushion, my heart still aches, and I am not sure I can come to terms with being a childless couple. It is so hard when you truly believe that it has happened, that the cycle worked. All the little signs of potential pregnancy and then the hard reality when the blue line appears on its own, and just like that it's over.

***

Weeks go by and we don't really discuss anything. The emotional wounds show a little and we give each other a look every now and then. One day out of the blue a medical appointment comes through the door. I don't really pass much remarks on it. I put the letter on the sideboard, pop the kettle on and call for Keith.

'Hey, how was work?' I call.

I casually open my letters and discover the medical one is from the regional fertility clinic and we have an appointment to commence our treatment. I am shaking with nerves and shock. I look at Keith to see his reaction, and he is looking at me for mine. It is one of those moments that you never forget, like where you were when JKF died. This is our one and only paid cycle. Our government allows one on the health care system. We have waited four years for this. Imagine four years ago we started this journey, and we are only starting this one. We should be elated. Instead we are tired, emotionally and physically drained. I cry. I cry hard. I am not sure why, but that's what came out—tears. Knowing I have to do this, there is no choice and we have to go right back to the start. Now that might sound selfish, but fear was the ultimate emotion. Fear of everything, the intrusive tests, the injections, the hiding, the rollercoaster and ultimately, it not working.

I gather my thoughts, and we arrange dinner. I don't say much because I don't know how I am feeling. I take a bath and have an early night. I sleep like a baby and wake up the next morning with a newfound excitement and enthusiasm for the journey. It won't be the same. It is a new journey, new consultants and a whole new plan with more information from the last two failed cycles. I have a tilted uterus, and we need to make sure they know. I do not know if this is relevant, but I will surely mention it. Keith is relieved I've woken like this and says he didn't really know what to say yesterday as he was delighted, and my reaction took him back. I laughed as hard as I have in ages and realise this is what I am meant to do and it's our journey.

I phone the appointment line and make an appointment for two weeks. We have to travel to the city again and start from the beginning. I remind Keith he has to play his part again, and he fills with dread. Even though I may feel I have the majority to do, I also recognise Keith has a vital role to play, and he goes through this all with me emotionally.

***

The two weeks go by quickly, and we are back down the road again. Same towns, same fields and same hopes surface. It is a lovely time of year. Spring has arrived. Leaves are growing on the trees, and it is time for another chance. I like to think everything has meaning, and this feels right. I am a little concerned about this meeting. It is like a book-in meeting, the initial one where everything has to be questioned, forms have to be filled in and more tests. I am afraid I have been comfort eating since the last failed attempt and my BMI might be too high. It is the silly things that distract you. We are not in the main hospital. We are at some health centre, a little on the other side of the city. The receptionist greets us as we walk in. She is friendly and books us in. We walk up a long corridor and take our seats. We are brought in together initially to discuss our fertility issues and again answer all the questions. It is funny at this stage as the consultant is the spitting image of a president who was in power at the time. It is actually uncanny. Keith and I just glance at each other, knowing what each other is thinking. He has our medical notes from previous meetings and why the referral was made and the results from years ago when we were at the investigation stage.

A nurse comes in and takes me to another room. I am weighed, all was ok there, I am not sure why I worried. I then have to give blood, take embarrassing swabs and discuss my menstrual cycle in intimate detail. I have kept a diary as I had to previously. The detail needs to be as accurate as possible to ensure treatment is optimum to give the best chance. I go back into the room and the consultant talks over our potential plan. He suggests going for ICSI again. This is because of the results of the tests we underwent some time ago. We explain that in between times we have had two failed cycles. He asks lots of questions about that and we tell him about the over stimulation, how our embryos were frozen and about the tilted uterus that appeared to complicate the transfer process. I had brought our previous schedule to show and any

91

details I felt necessary. He asked if it was ok for him to access our file from the private clinic. We agreed anything that would help us on this journey was worth having. He discussed our previous cycles and writes this all down. He also agrees to do a trial run of the insemination to ensure the angle is right at the time of procedure. We talk about the medication and possibility of commencing soon. We are sent along our way and for me to track my cycle. Now we have had this meeting and providing all tests are fine, we will start soon. We leave the office once again full of hope. There is a café in the health centre, so we go there to have a cup of tea and a bite to eat before heading down the road home. There is a pool at the centre, and we watch people swimming lengths of the pool.

'That seemed to go well,' I say once we are settled and the evitable conversation comes up about the look alike status of our consultant. We need to keep things light-hearted as this journey is so intense. I know from the past you can get lost in it. The food is edible, and we go for a short walk around the area when we are there. We are in no rush home, and it is a lovely day.

Again, we decide not to tell anyone for the same reasons as before. This seems to be happening promptly after so many years. This suits us both. Work is going well, and I do not foresee any big in-house events coming up, so hopefully my role will be non-eventful for the next while. Well, as uneventful as a journalist can be.

Keith and I discuss our expectations and talk about if we'd waited four years for this appointment and not went private, we would not have all the information we have now. Thankfully, the consultant is taking it on.

We plan a little trip, some *us* time before it all starts. We decide to fly off to somewhere hot and just relax by the pool for a few days. This was a welcomed break and a great time to reconnect. This is so important throughout this journey. With the sun on my face and a slight breeze, I watch families play in the pool. Lots of laughter, some tears and plenty of noise. Keith jumps in full of excitement and I lounge round the pool taking in the vitamin D. I cannot swim, so the pool does not interest me much. I enjoy reading and people watching. We go for long walks and eat lovely food. Feeling rejuvenated, we are ready to take on this rollercoaster we are about to embark.

Keith's job has changed a bit, and he is now working with new people. This is a welcomed distraction, and we meet up a few times over the next few weeks. They invited us down to their home in the secluded surroundings of mountains. We accept the offer with no commitment to dates as we do not know what lies ahead for us. Hoping this doesn't seem rude, but these are the things you have to weave around while going through the process and sacrifices that have to be made. I am happy for them to think I am being awkward. After all, they do not know me or what we are going through. People should not judge. You truly never know what people are going through. I call to see Mum. She's happy as always spring has arrived, and she is out in the garden. I bring her back a souvenir from holidays keeping with tradition. This is a fan as she likes to collect them, the more colourful the better. I tell her of the wonderful time we had, and she comments on the nice glow I have from the sun. I ensure she has all that she needs, and I head home. It is always nice to see Mum and just sit and chat for a while.

The girls call as I haven't seen them since our holiday, and they are keen to catch up. I agree to connect, and we all meet up for a coffee, kids in tow, and it is great. The girls are busy asking questions about my holiday, the flight, the food, sandy beaches and they're envious of my carefree lifestyle or so it appears. And here they are with children running around and making noise, looking for attention and stuffing their little faces and I love it. Funny how there is a different perspective on things. My life is really good. I have no complaints. I just feel incomplete. I want to bear a child. I want Keith's child to complete our family. The ache is real.

Chapter 9

Round Three

My cycle tracked and paperwork complete, the hospital has been informed and our next appointment is on the way. I am feeling hopeful again, even though I promised myself not to be. I have set the intention, so where attention goes energy flows. I am full of positive intention and an unwavering knowing that this will work. So, I meditate again, this time mindful meditation and walking meditation, which is new for me. I can feel myself getting sucked into the bubble again and need to keep external interests going too. Work is always a good distraction and I cannot believe it when another smaller project comes up to allow me to completely immerse myself. I again have to ask my manager for days off and perhaps a few mornings, though with this new project he says it might be tight. I try not to let this worry me too much and remind myself to take it a day at a time. No stress. I ponder where it all went wrong the last two times. Did I not lie for long enough afterwards? Is the journey too much? Am I stressed? Am I eating the right foods? There are a thousand reasons to why and no answers.

Back down the road again. It is another lovely day. We leave in plenty of time and stop at our usual garage for coffee and tea, a banana and some chocolate. Such creatures of habit. Our appointment is for late morning and we are glad so we can get up and head there straight away. We listen to a podcast in the car. I doze in between sessions. I find being a passenger hard sometimes and I probably did not sleep too well last night. The city isn't too bad, and we have to go to the other side, or so I thought. When we arrive, we are early, so we just stroll around. When I go to the desk with my letter, the lady tells me there is no clinic today. There must be a misunderstanding. I look at the letter again, and we are definitely the right time and day. The lady lifts the phone and phones across to the booking line at the main hospital and informs us that we are at the wrong place. We should be at the main hospital fertility clinic and not back at the same centre as before. Keith and I look at each other in panic and the lady asks if we can still attend our appointment but we are at the other end of the city and will be awhile. My heart is beating so fast because if we miss this appointment, we might miss the whole month as everything is so timed. The lady gets off the phone and tells us to head over to the main hospital. They know that we are coming and will wait for us. We dash to the car and sit in silence. The letter did not state a building, and I just assumed it was the same as before. What a start to our journey? This is the type of stress we can do without.

When we finally get there, the car park is full. We have to drive round and round. Keith asks if I want to get out and go in first and he will find a space, but I refuse as it is the first time. I want us to go in together. We eventually get parked and head over to the main building. The fertility clinic was easy to find as there is a huge sign outside. We go in to the first doors and wait for the receptionist to take our name and let us in. It is all very clinical, white walls, strange floor tiles, uncomfortable seats. We sit to the back. The room is full; I mean absolutely full of couples, some young, others are older. You can feel the hope in the room. I take a moment to take it all in. This is huge. All these couples are the same as us and somewhere on the same journey. I turn to Keith with a look of disbelief. I just sit back. Keith takes out his phone and takes a picture of us. He sends it to me with a caption, 'this is going to work.' Which was the right thing to say at the exact right time. We have to wait sometime before being called but I don't mind as we were lucky to be taken at all. When we go in, the nurse see us first. She takes my weight again and sits us down for a chat. She explains what will happen today, a little about the timeline and about the consultant. I am familiar with some of the terminology and we are happy going forward. She then takes us down into another room to meet the consultant. This is a much smaller room and again very clinical. I notice baby photos all over the board with thank you captions. This fills me with joy and a visual of what can and has been achieved. The consultant notices me looking.

He says, 'We will have your little ones picture up there some day.'

I smile from ear to ear, so happy with the thought.

We discuss my cycle, our previous treatment attempts. The consultant now has the file from the private clinic. He looks over the schedule and discusses his thoughts on the best way forward. Then he makes some decisions based on the over stimulation of my ovaries and my tilted pelvis which he feels is no issue and quite common. He wants to do a trial run of the transfer and note down the best insertion route. I am pleased to hear this even though it means coming back down for a trial run and of course the uncomfortableness of the procedure. I feel listened to here and understood, which is a great relief and less stressful. I am not sure if it is because we have been down this road before or the genuine nature of the staff. I suspect it is the staff, their obvious commitment for this to be successful. We discuss the treatment plan or schedule as they call it in detail. It seems to be a lower dose for longer. We are going for ICSI again and need to take over my cycle, stimulate my ovaries and trigger ovulation so they can retrieve my eggs. It is all very controlled and timed to perfection. The consultant writes me out a prescription for all the medication I need. Keith and I leave the fertility centre and go to the main hospital to the pharmacy department. I hand in my prescription and wait. It is busy, and lots of people are coming and going. I sit and people watch. There are all kinds of people. Some who look particularly unwell, some in wheelchairs and others who do not look too bad.

My mind wonders of the volume of people who come through the doors daily and how unwell some people are. I truly count my blessings and feel grateful for the opportunity to try again. My name is called, and I walk up to the screen. I am handed a rather big blue bag of medication. I am a little taken back by the amount that appears to be in the bag. The feeling of complete dread comes over me and a reminder of the injections and the impact they had on me. I smile and signal to Keith to come on, and we leave the room. I do not say much as I am a little overwhelmed. Keith carries the bag for me, and we head back to meet the consultant as he now has the schedule printed out for me. He also wants to check the contents of the bag to ensure everything is correct. Everything is in the bag, all the injections for stimulation, the trigger, the yellow box that is the needle dispenser and the suppositories along with a leaflet and some guidance. Once the contents are checked, we then discuss the schedule. It is a little different than last time but laid out on the page better. The last time it was like an Excel document. This time it is simple, the days and dates are set out on it and it makes more sense. Sometimes it is the simple things that really help along the way. Just like that we are leaving with everything we need to get the process started to hopefully have our own baby.

We drive home and stop at a restaurant just outside the city. We decide it is better to make our way to our end of the city and in the direction of home. At least then we will not be panicking and enjoy our lunch. These are all the lessons we have learnt from the previous times.

Back home all is well, and we just relax. I am a little nervous about the injections again and excited also feelings of hope are back again, but the meditation is helping me stay focussed. Keith and I meditate together. We even have a mantra now. We thought it might help a positive outcome, and also it is a lovely thing to do together.

***

Up and back at it. Work is always a welcome distraction. Our new community project is a lovely one, working with community and voluntary groups delivering an eight-week course. We are partners in the project and are expected to attend every session. They start at 10am every Tuesday for eight weeks. *This will be fun.* Hopefully, I do not have to head to the city on a Tuesday. I will check the dates when I get home. It also depends on stimulation. I am not too worried. I will work something out should it arise.

Back down the road to the city for my mock transfer. It is not a nice experience but necessary to ensure nothing stops the embryologist from a straightforward transfer. Keith comes too, although I said he did not have to, but he felt he wanted to for support me as he cannot attend all of my scan appointments during the stimulation process. Keith appears a little nervous. I reach over to hold his hand and give reassurance. Parking is a nightmare as usual and we have learnt to go high up the stories to get a space. We are back in the same building seeing our consultant. We do not have to wait long; the nurse calls me in. I have to gown up and go to the clinical theatre room for the mock procedure. Keith comes too. I wait in the room. The consultant comes in, explains what will happen and asks the nurse to write down his directions. I get myself into position, and the consultant completes the procedure. He explains he is happy with everything, and the nurse takes notes to ensure a smooth transition. We thank him and leave. Another thing done on our journey. I am not that hungry and ask Keith to go straight home. I am a bit niggly after the procedure and want to relax. I am aware I will see this road many more times over the next few weeks.

Ok, so here we go first day of injections. I ensure I've placed all the vials in the fridge. The liquid is cold when I take it out. I ask Keith to check the dosage and help me draw up the first one just to refresh my memory and give me a little confidence doing it. The bottles are a little different than last time and the amount. Eek! It stings, but all is well. *I can do this. I have done it before and I can do this*; I tell myself. That sting, the mental attitude to keep pushing through the sting and the pain. Having to watch as the liquid of the injection enters my body. Trying not to rush it and at the same time wanting to hurry up to get it over and done with. My whole body tenses, which does not help my tummy, still traumatised from the last cycle and the little red pin holes still visible. I already feel the intensity of the injections and am reminded of the impact of the last times

I have my dates to attend the clinic for my scans and check-ups, and of course, two of them are on Tuesdays. Typical, but all is not lost. They are at 8am in the morning. It takes two hours to get through the city. Traffic will not be too bad so I may be a little late for my project session, but that all good too. The injections are going as well as can be expected. I have put on a little weight since the last two attempts and I have a little tummy. This may help with the injections. I still chew chewing gum when doing them. It distracts me or helps with the pain; I am not sure which. I am battling through them, regardless. My emotions are all over the place again. I am preoccupied with my thoughts and trying hard not to be.

I get up at 5am and pack myself a little breakfast and snack to eat in the car. I won't stop on the way, and I will not have time on the way back. I say goodbye to Keith, who cannot come because of work commitments. I leave in plenty of time as I am on my own and do not want any stress. I play music loudly the whole way there. I love music and playing it for two hours straight as loud as I want is heaven, Pink being the artist of choice. When I arrive, I check in at the door and I am buzzed in as I walk through the doors. I take a breath; the room is full, full of couples waiting. *What is going on?* So many people need support with their fertility, and they are of all different ages. Surely this cannot be right. Fertility issues are more common than people realise and, being a journalist, I research this specifically to my region and then wider areas. It's unbelievable this is such a problem with limited funding from the government and very few resources to highlight the issue. It is so taboo. Admittedly, I have kept it a secret too, though my reasons are because I do not want to be mollycoddled. I need to stay strong and I do this best on my own.

I am called by the nurse and have my check up and scan. All is well, not too much happening as it is still early in the treatment cycle. They want me back more regularly than previously discussed to ensure I do not overstimulate. I really hope this does not happen as I am hoping for a fresh transfer. There is not much difference in success between a fresh and frozen transfer, it is about getting to blastocyst stage, which is important. I would just prefer to keep going, however, what will be will be. I am happy with the process so far and head back down the road. I listen to music and snack in the car. Keith phones and I update him. I make it to the venue of the project about ten minutes late and no one really passes much remarks. I am glad of this as I have to go back next week. I am feeling rather proud of myself, like I can achieve anything. A whole process of fertility treatment and still work throughout it. The morning passes quickly, and it is relaxing. Just what I need after a 5am start and a four-hour round trip. The bright mornings help. I get to see the sunrise and feel the start of the day a new dawn.

***

We have been asked by Keith's friends to visit this weekend. Keith says yes, and I am a little reluctant as I am in the middle of our treatment cycle and I do not want anything to happen or any upset. Keith convinces me it is a good idea and a welcome distraction and oh yeah, we are climbing a mountain, so sort of team building exercise. I assure Keith I am definitely not climbing any mountain. Although there would probably be no reason not to, I do not like taking any chances. One more clinic appointment over and we are packed up and ready for a two-hour trip the opposite direction to Keith's colleague / friend's house. I am a little nervous as I have to bring my injections with me. I remind Keith I have to take them at the same time and do not want to defer from this.

We have a lovely drive. It is very scenic. I have never been down this part of the country before. We drive through a national park, and the mountain we are meant to climb. I make a joke about Keith having fun climbing the mountain. He does not think it is as funny as I do. We finally arrive and are made to feel welcome. We freshen up and head for something to eat. I offer to drive as I am not drinking and that allows for the rest to relax and have a wee tipple. We have a lovely evening, and everyone gets on well, lots of laughter and fun, just what we need. I get up early and prepare for my injection. It still stings, and my tummy is surely a pin cushion at this stage. Keith is fast asleep, so I inject in the room. I even brought the yellow box to dispense of the needle. We get up, and it is raining so no mountain climb for the group. I think everyone is happy enough though. Keith and I head into the small village along with the group. We have a walk around and visit some sights and do a little souvenir shopping. It is a lovely village. We can see what the tourist attraction would be. We head back to the house and say our goodbyes. I want to get home for the next injection and lie up and relax. I am tired of travelling at this stage. I feel I have supported Keith well this weekend, and he seems genuinely pleased with his new work colleagues.

They say a Sunday well spent brings a week of content and I take this on board and prepare for the week ahead. I wash and iron all my outfits for the week, nothing too tight to my tummy for comfort. I cook meals for seven days. I freeze some and refrigerate the others. It is probably more to do with nerves than being organised, but I know it will make the week ahead a lot easier.

***

Tuesday and back down the road again. I pack breakfast and a little snack. Nutrition is so important, especially throughout this treatment. I arrive once again to a packed room of hopeful couples all aiming for the same outcome. Unfortunately, statistically speaking, many of us will be disappointed, though the sheer volume of people in the room speaks for itself. My appointment goes well, and the eggs are growing well in my ovaries. I am given another appointment for two days' time and they say I may soon be triggering ovulation. I am happy all is going well. I head back down the road, phone Keith with the update and go straight in to work from the appointment.

It is a strange feeling when stimulating the ovaries through the treatment as you can feel something is happening like a tightening of your ovaries felt in your tummy. Perhaps I am just very aware of it, but I can definitely feel it happening. After work, I head home. Keith is there preparing one of the precooked meals. I am grateful for this. *I should do this every Sunday.* Then reality hits and I realise that probably won't happen. Sundays are a precious reset day usually, only I was so aware of the week ahead, I got organised.

Keith comes to the next appointment and they measure my follicles. Everyone seems happy, and I am given the date to trigger ovulation through the HCG injection. I am excited as no over stimulation has happened and hopefully won't in between times. Keith and I arrange days off for the next week as the egg retrieval will happen. They use a strong pain relief and I will be drowsy and after the last time I felt unwell, so we are taking no chances. We are also well aware that if all goes well at the egg retrieval and insemination is successful, we will aim for the transfer six days later if we make it to blastocyst. The nurse writes down instructions of times and dates for trigger and when to come for egg retrieval and semen sample. All systems go. We stop for food on the way home and take in the news of what will happen over the next few days. You have to take each stage as it comes even though we know what will happen. We learnt that the first time. Still, we are hopeful, and you can see it in our eyes.

I keep myself busy over the next couple of days, though I do not go visiting or make contact except my daily phone call to Mum. I am one of those people who you can see in my face if something is going on, so I avoid contact just to keep myself well.

It is good we have been to this point before it's prepared us for the procedures. We are however hopeful for smooth retrieval and no complications. We get up early. I have packed a comfort bag for the journey and in the recovery room for after. I am feeling calm and Keith looks calm which is good, and we leave in plenty of time. We have an early appointment so do not expect much traffic. We got a good parking space and head into the clinic and we are called straight away by the nurse for book in. Keith is taken to another room to play his part, and I am gowned and ready to go. Keith comes out just before I go in and reassures me. I am brought into the theatre. The embryologist comes in and the nurse checks my details to make sure all is correct. I am given some pain killers which make me very drowsy, and really; I remember very little. The next thing I know I am being wheeled out to Keith into the recovery room. I am lying on the bed. We are in a room with about five bays with beds and a curtain dividing us. There is a girl next to us crying her heart out because they only retrieved two eggs and she is very upset as she feels her chances are limited. Keith and I recognise after our last two cycles that having lots of eggs does not mean that you have a better chance. All you need is that one high quality embryo that takes and it only takes one.

The nurse comes out and gives us the news that we have twelve. This is a lot less than last time but then again, I over stimulated and there were lots of eggs. We are happy, and the nurse appears pleased. It is not what we had before, but it is definitely enough for us. I lie another while and have some tea. The nurse comes back and say we can leave now if I am feeling all right and someone from the lab will phone tomorrow with an update on insemination and fertilisation. We are happy to leave and head home. As I am tired and feeling a little tender and nauseous, we don't stop. We are feeling excited and relieved that all to this stage has gone well. We have eggs, which is amazing, and I have no more injections. Now just to wait for updates on the eggs hoping they fertilise, and embryos are created. There is no place like home. When we get there, I take a shower, put comfy clothes on, get a blanket and lie on the sofa. Keith organises food and we just relax the rest of the day.

I have taken the next day off work. Keith has to go to work so I just lie in bed, flicking through my phone. I try to consciously think about the fertilisation process and imagine good, healthy grade A embryos. I visualise them growing and becoming strong. Hopefully, somewhere in the lab new life is beginning. A little after lunchtime, the phone rings and it is the embryologist ringing to say we have nine embryos. Three had not taken and the nine look strong. They have them back in the incubator and will ring in two days, which will be day three. I am happy with the result and phone Keith. We are both excited and apprehensive. It is an emotional rollercoaster, and we just have to trust the process at this stage. Waiting on the call over the next two days is hard. I try to occupy myself. It works a little, but I can't help wondering if they are growing and splitting and forming well. The gift of life truly is a miracle. When you really think about the process, it is an amazing thing. We are all cells and how we come to be. It is only when you have to think about it so much and understand the process, do you really take it in. It is the most natural thing in the world we just need a helping hand.

'Day three embryos,' the embryologist says on the phone. 'Each one is looking favourable, some more than others. They are aiming to get to blastocyst.'

I reply I am happy to wait for that even if it means some dropping off as blastocyst is a good starting point for insemination and for the embryo to take. Keith is with me when I get the call as it is the weekend. I write an email to my boss asking for next week off as it will be embryo transfer day and I want to take it easy after. I should have asked before now, though I was waiting to see how I was feeling and did not want to assume we would get to this part.

***

It is embryo transfer day. We have to leave early, so I organised the night before. I have a bag packed for me, a pillow and blanket in the car for afterwards, snacks and a lunch for Keith. We are both feeling nervous as we have been here before and no baby yet. 'We need to believe,' I tell Keith, 'or else why are we doing this?'

We drive towards the sunrise. It is a beautiful day. The dew is still on the fields, and I am mindfully taking in the morning. We stop for our usual snacks. I cannot take them, but just to settle Keith's nerves, I am happy to stop. There is no traffic into the city as it is so early, and we get a parking space no problem. *So far, so good*, I think to myself.

We book in when we arrive and are taken through. The room is not so full this morning yet. It must be only those who have made it to this stage are in this morning, a stark reminder that not everyone gets here. I feel gratitude once again. I gown up as does Keith. This is a surgical procedure, everything is sterilised, and it is in a procedure room. I lie on the bed and take in my surroundings, nothing fancy. Some equipment looks old-fashioned. It is a dark room with a door to the left. The nurse comes in and checks my details. The embryologist comes in to say hello. It is a different person; someone we have not met before. This makes me nervous as it may be tricky to get the catheter where it needs to go. He doesn't really speak too much.

He says, 'Hello.'

The consultant is gowned up. He speaks to the nurses in the room. On the door to the left is where our beautiful little blastocysts are. We all again confirm name, date of birth and so on. This is now to ensure the right embryos are being transferred into the tube and then to me. I get into position and wait for the embryologist to come forward. He uses an ultrasound scanner on my tummy and on my lower back. This position is awkward, but I do not care. I just want a successful transfer. The nurse holds the ultrasound equipment in place. The embryologist takes the tube from the other embryologist and comes forward. He asks me to tilt a little. Keith is sitting beside me. We are watching the screen. We can see the tube going in and the transfer taking place and just at that, a flash of white light. I smile and say, 'Did you see that?'

The nurse and Keith both confirm they see the same. It was a surreal moment. I never experienced anything like it in my life.

The embryologist takes the catheter out and says, 'Ok. that's us then. I wish you all the best for a successful pregnancy.'

He appeared sure of himself. He didn't speak much and in fact was quick. We could tell he was obviously experienced at this. The nurse advised me to lie for a moment as I'd my legs up high. I need to lie straight for a moment before sitting upright. There is no waiting around after. It is perfectly safe to get up and go on, but I like to lie for a few minutes hoping nature has now taken over and the embryo has taken.

After I get dressed and sorted the nurse gives me a pack. It contains suppositories and a pregnancy test with a leaflet on guidance on when to take the test and how to insert the suppositories. They are the same as the last ones and are very important to take helping nature on its way.

Keith and I walk out the double doors of the clinic and down the path. We look at each other, and say that's worked, we could just feel it. The embryologist appeared so confident and sure, and the white light! Oh my goodness, what an experience! I am still amazed by it.

I am feeling all right, but I lie in the back seat covered in the blanket. I eat a snack and Keith listens to a podcast the whole way home. I do not mind the transfer so much; it is the egg retrieval that is hard I feel because of the whole procedure and also feeling nauseous and drowsy after.

***

We are now into the summer months, and it is a beautiful warm day when we get home. I open all the windows and go to bed for a while. I am tired emotionally and physically. What a rollercoaster and it is not over yet. We have the dreaded two-week wait. This is hard as I watch every move, every niggle and ache. I have been here twice before and feel a little more settled. We head to the beach for the day as we live near a seaside town. We go for a walk along the beach. It is lovely to feel the sun on my face and the sand between my toes. I have a sense of achievement that we made it through another treatment cycle. I still feel tender and I am being kind to myself. My tummy is still like a pincushion. The good thing about summer is I can wear loose dresses. It is not that my tummy is sore. It's just tender and feels a little swollen from the inside after the transfer. We go for something to eat and just enjoy the day. Sea air is amazing. It makes you feel alive and watching the sea is so calming. We get home and empty the car. There is sand everywhere and Keith hoovers it immediately. I phone Mum to say hi and tell her about our day. Nothing special, but another day closer to test day.

I'm feeling good, a little distracted preoccupied with my thoughts. It is ten days now since the transfer, and I am feeling unsettled. I go upstairs and into our room and take out the test. I cannot help myself; I want to do it. Without telling Keith, I take the test. I pee in a bottle and dip the stick in. The test is a funny-looking test, not like shop bought ones. I wait and wait, pacing the bathroom floor. I set my alarm for two minutes and wait for the buzzer. The phone buzzes and I take a deep breath, I lift the test and look, and there it is, two blue lines.

TWO BLUE LINES!

I can hardly breathe. I throw the door open and scream as best I can for Keith. He does not know what is going on and comes running.

'What? Are you all right?' he asks.

'Keith, Keith, it has worked,' I say. 'We are having a baby,' I explain while standing on top of the stairs shaking. Keith starts to shake too.

'Wait, what?'

I try to get the words out to tell him I have taken the test, and it is positive. I hand him the test and the guidance paper. We cannot believe it. We hug each other, shaking with disbelief and excitement. Is it real? Is it right? We are elated and in disbelief. Keith goes into the local supermarket and buys two more tests. It is early in the morning with not many about, so he is happy to go. I wait for Keith to come back, just sitting, taking it all in. I'm pregnant. I look back at the test again and there are definitive two blue lines. When Keith comes back, I take another test, and it comes back positive immediately. I am tempted to take another one but leave it until I was supposed to take it. For now, and at this moment in time, we are having a baby. I am pregnant. We sit on the sofa and just take it in, the journey, the ups and the downs and now we have a positive test. A little baby is growing inside of me. We touch my tummy and hold it for a moment to recognise our baby is in there.

Life goes on as normal. We go to work as usual, but nothing is normal. We are having a baby. I admit I have a smirk on my face all day. Nothing takes my focus off the fact I am pregnant. Everyone at work notices I am different somehow but put it down to me having a wonderful week off work with Keith and being relaxed. *If only they knew.* We will not tell anyone until twelve weeks. We agreed that after we took the test, although we had spoken about it on occasions before.

On the official day of the two-week wait, I take another test. I feel a little nervous again, doubts enter my head. I pee on the stick, set my alarm and wait. It's all a waiting game. Again, we have a positive test. I feel so happy, so grateful and appreciate the health care we have received that got us to this point. I remember the flash of white light at the transfer and believe this was our beautiful baby. I phone the number on the leaflet to confirm the result. The nurse congratulates us and gives us a date to come down for the confirmation scan. It is a few weeks away, but I am content with that. Wow, what a journey so far. It is strange knowing so early that we are pregnant. We even know to the exact moment of conception. These will be great stories for the grandkids. Keith and I laugh about it. We are getting ahead of ourselves now. We are so excited it is hard to contain. It's true! We are going to be parents. Our two will become three. Our family will be complete.

Chapter 10

Scan Day

It is scan day. We officially book in our pregnancy. We have to go back to the city to the regional fertility clinic to confirm it is a viable pregnancy and we are so excited. At this stage we will be four weeks pregnant. I have to drink water to help with the scan. This is harder than it seems, as with a two-hour journey I would need the toilet before we got there. We think of the practicalities, and I do not drink lots of water until we get there as we will arrive early to allow time for this. We stop on the way for our usual coffee, tea, chocolate and banana. It was poignant as it may be our last trip to the city during this journey as hopefully, they will direct us to our local hospital from now on, all being well. We arrive in good time. I am full of water and hoping I can last. We check in, and the nurse takes us down to a room for our scan. The excitement is real. I lie on the bed and pull down my bottoms to the pelvic bone. She squirts cold gel on my tummy. She rolls the scanner over my tummy. We cannot see the screen at this stage. She asks questions about dates and when we took the test. I feel a little nervous as she is not giving anything away. She confirms she has located the sac and is measuring it. The nurse then leaves the room. Keith and I are then left worrying if everything is all right. We haven't been given an indication that anything is wrong, though no reassurance either. The nurse comes back with a consultant, and he then scans my tummy.

'Ok, yes,' he says.

They turn the screen around so we can see.

'Ok,' he says. 'Here we are. Here is your baby, and it is measuring ok. And here also is another baby.'

'Oh my goodness,' we say.

'I never thought of two, to be honest.'

'Yes,' the nurse says.

She needed the consultant to come in to confirm as they are not the same size. One is smaller than the other, but there is definitely two. One is progressing better than the other is really what they said. They congratulate us both and print us a photograph of the scan. We then have to fill out some forms and the nurse wishes us well and asks up to keep them updated in progress. I remember the photographs on the wall and say I cannot wait until our babies are up on the wall. We are now referred to our local hospital and we say our goodbyes. Our journey to the city has ended, and all being well, we will be under the care of our local maternity unit.

Twins! We are having twins. What a surprise this time round. I had not even thought of the possibility. It is still early days. We are only four weeks in, and we are aware of that. I phone my GP to book into my practice and they've sent the referral to our local hospital. Everything is falling into place.

***

The weeks go by and we tell our families we are expecting a baby. Everyone is delighted. Some people are shocked as they thought we were choosing not to have children. I have informed work. Most importantly, I think I am feeling flutters. I am so in tune with my body given all that we have been through. Everything is going well. We have our fifteen-week scan. It is supposed to be twelve weeks, but the waiting times are high, it is fifteen weeks before we are seen. I am ok with this because we have already seen the babies. Well, one definite progressive pregnancy and the other was not as progressive. Surely if I had lost one, I would have had a physical reaction and it would be obvious. We are at our local hospital and it is much easier not to travel to the regional fertility clinic. They felt we were low risk for complications, so were happy for us to go mainstream and so are we. We have to book in and answer a lot of questions at this appointment. They take bloods, my blood pressure and weight. Then on to meet the consultant to say hello and have a scan. We are so excited. This is a big scan and I have to drink a lot beforehand, so it is easier to see the babies.

I lie on the bed, Keith by my side, and wait for the consultant. The nurse lays out a tissue on my clothes and then comes the cold gel. The consultant rolls the scanner around my tummy and we can see a large circle with movement inside. He explains the outline, and what everything is. Tears fill our eyes as we can now see an outline of a baby. The consultant carefully moves the scanner around for the second baby. I am no expert at scans, but I knew if it was taking so long, it wasn't good. The consultant informs us that is he sorry but there is only one active pregnancy. He shows us the empty sac where life had once begun, but not progressed. We are a little upset but do not say much. We are so pleased and thankful for our wonderful healthy baby on the scan. They wipe my tummy and print us another picture. We are so proud we can see our little baby and in the background of the picture you can make out the empty sac which I like so it wasn't forgotten. Being through fertility treatment, I recognise the baby from the insemination. And embryos grow as we have been aware every step of the way, and prayed for growing embryos, seeing each one as a baby at the start of life.

Keith goes on back to work and I am brought into the midwives' room to collect my file and discuss pregnancy, especially being a first-time mum. This is a great opportunity to discuss any concerns I have. It is here that I break down and cry for the second baby that did not make it. Silly to some, but the loss was very upsetting to me.

'Where did it go?' I ask. 'I never felt anything and where will the empty sac go now?'

The midwife spent loads of time reassuring and comforting me with all my questions.

I leave with my green file. I have to take it to all my appointments, some in my GP practice and some with the hospital. When I get to the car, I phone Mum and start to cry. Mum doesn't know what is wrong. I eventually blurt out the baby is grand, I have a picture, but there is only one. Mum is sympathetic even though we had been given information that one was progressing and the other potentially not. It is only when you see it and are told for sure that you really take it in.

I go home and have a cup of tea. Keith rings and we chat about the baby that did not make it and get excited about our beautiful baby on the way. Keith videoed the scan and is convinced the baby is waving at him. It is lovely to see Keith get excited and feel more involved. We buy a Doppler so we can hear the heartbeat all the time and so Keith can be part of every step. Keith sings 'Everyday' by Buddy Holly to my ever-growing tummy, connecting to the baby at a deep level. I am so pleased about this as it can be hard for dads. I feel the connection already. My love for our child is already there, and I have never felt like this in my life. We have decided not to find out the sex of the baby and be old-fashioned and wait until the birth, so everything is yellow or green. I do not want to buy too much until the baby arrives safely and all is well. We have yearned for so long for our baby. It still seems too good to be true. The miracle of life is amazing. We celebrate Christmas and the New Year in real parents-to-be style. Everything was about waiting for our new addition. It's January now, with big changes to our lives. We are really looking forward to this year. I am feeling a little breathless most of the time and any long distance is uncomfortable for me.

The girls and I decide an evening out is on the cards and we book a restaurant for early January to avoid the Christmas rush. We go to our local Greek restaurant and have a lovely evening. Upon leaving I bump into Neill, my colleague who I met after the first failed cycle. I am quite big, and he congratulates me on my pregnancy. Little does he know he played a part in the journey. Perhaps I will tell him some day. The girls are gushing over me, asking if I will find out the sex of the baby or if I had seen on the scan. They are so excited for me and for us as a group of friends. We have now renamed ourselves the yummy mummies. Very fitting, I feel.

***

Over the next few weeks I am rushed by ambulance into hospital with a suspected clot because of my breathlessness and raised blood pressure. I am kept in for observation and tests and given a clexitine injection. More injections in my tummy, this time to stop or dispel a clot. A week in hospital has been such a fright and to think if anything happened to the baby would just be devastating. They have signed me off work and told to rest. Just over two months to go now. I am resting up and getting bigger by the day. The breathlessness is still here, but manageable. I attend GP and hospital appointments weekly to keep an eye on me and the baby when I take a turn for the worst. My left leg swells, and my breathing significantly worsens. I am admitted to hospital for more tests and treatment. My due date is ten days away, and they consider inducing me. They are reluctant and are happy to keep me for observation. I am in the safest place. Not what we wanted for the end of our pregnancy, but all is well.

A lady consultant comes in on a Friday evening. I ask can I go home just to make sure everything is ready for the baby's arrival and so I can rest properly. We only live ten minutes away, which is within the safe zone in terms of emergency. She gets my file, and we discuss our options. I also explain we are having an ICSI baby and know the exact day of conception and if the baby does not come beforehand, can we be induced on our due date? This would mean we have gone full term and not allow for any compilations going past the due date. She checks the schedule and delivers the good news that I can go home for the weekend and come back on Monday morning for induction on Tuesday. We are delighted, and this gives us the weekend to prepare. I bounce up and down on a Pilates ball all weekend trying to bring on some movement and entice the baby to come, but nothing worked.

Monday morning has arrived. I am so nervous for what is ahead of me. I am grateful to have got this far. I made the mistake of watching birthing videos on the internet and have spooked myself. When we arrive, they take us downstairs and meet some of the midwives. Everyone is lovely. I am booked in and given some gel to see if that might start labour. They move us up to the birthing ward, a lovely big room. If I was to go myself, the baby will be delivered here. I bounce and bounce on the birthing ball they have. I spend most of the day on the phone with well-wishers and people texting. I have brought a book in with me. I imagine I was a sight to behold bouncing on a ball with my tummy nearly as big as the ball facing the window reading a book. The nurses and midwives call in throughout the day and evening, hoping for some signs of labour, but nothing is happening. We are waiting for me to dilate. Keith goes home. He appears very lonesome and a little nervous. I walk him to the end of the corridor. We hug, and he leaves. It is late, and I promise to phone him straight away if anything happens.

The next day is the same. No movement and Keith and I are pacing the floors. I am getting niggles in my back. Surely that is something. The midwife comes in and checks me again and decides I am favourable to be brought to the labour ward. This is it. We are on our way. Keith is whiter than white. I change into a gown; they explain what will happen and about pain relief. Just like that I am in labour, and exactly two hours and thirty-five minutes later, our baby is born, all 9Lb 5OZ. The end was difficult. When she came out, the umbilical cord was around her neck leaving us with bated breath for what seemed like age, but was only two seconds. The midwives were amazing. They asked Keith to cut the cord. I look at Keith. He is a perfect shade of grey and really does not know what has just happened. He is really in shock. The midwives urge him to tell me what the baby is. They were so excited as they knew we did not know, and this normally does not happen. Keith looked at me and looked at the midwives with a confused look on his face. We all waited and Keith said, 'What is it? Is it a girl?'

To which the midwives were filled with delight and said, 'Yes.

Keith turned to me and said, 'It's a girl,' and just like that, the tears came. He was so happy. Lying there waiting, I opened my top, and they lay my beautiful daughter on my chest. A rush of emotion came over me and a feeling of love that I never thought possible filled me and I knew it was all worth it. My perfect baby girl had completed my family. My life and my heart were full.

About the Author

Emma Weaver is a member of the Everything Publishing Academy, this is Emma's first book one which came pouring out of her to reach out to people going through fertility challenges and treatment.

Her purpose in life is to advocate for appropriate support and services for those who need it within the mental health and wellbeing sector. She has over twenty year's experience working in the mental health and wellbeing sector. Emma is the founder of mental wealth International and also works as a manager within Inspire wellbeing group.

Motivated by her purpose Emma provides hope and support to others through both her professional and personal experiences.

Emma currently resides in county Fermanagh a beautiful rural county in Ireland. Although a native of Clones, Emma lives very close to her homestead. She is the mother to three beautiful children who are her world and inspiration every day.